theclinics.com

PEDIATRIC CLINICS
OF NORTH AMERICA

Pediatric Emergencies, Part II

GUEST EDITORS
Donald Van Wie, DO
Ghazala Q. Sharieff, MD
James E. Colletti, MD

April 2006 • Volume 53 • Number 2

SAUNDERS

An Imprint of Elsevier, Inc.
PHILADELPHIA   LONDON   TORONTO   MONTREAL   SYDNEY   TOKYO

W.B. SAUNDERS COMPANY

A Division of Elsevier Inc.

1600 John F. Kennedy Boulevard • Suite 1800 • Philadelphia, Pennsylvania 19103

http://www.theclinics.com

THE PEDIATRIC CLINICS OF NORTH AMERICA	Volume 53, Number 2
April 2006	ISSN 0031-3955
Editor: Carla Holloway	ISBN 1-4160-3655-5

The ideas and opinions expressed in *The Pediatric Clinics of North America* do not necessarily reflect those of the Publisher. The Publisher does not assume any responsibility for any injury and/or damage to persons or property arising out of or related to any use of the material contained in this periodical. The reader is advised to check the appropriate medical literature and the product information currently provided by the manufacturer of each drug to be administered to verify the dosage, the method and duration of administration, or contraindications. It is the responsibility of the treating physician or other health care professional, relying on independent experience and knowledge of the patient, to determine drug dosages and the best treatment for the patient. Mention of any product in this issue should not be construed as endorsement by the contributors, editors, or the Publisher of the product or manufacturers' claims.

The Pediatric Clinics of North America (ISSN 0031-3955) is published bi-monthly by W.B. Saunders, 360 Park Avenue South, New York, NY 10010-1710. Months of publication are February, April, June, August, October, and December. Business and Editorial Offices: 1600 John F. Kennedy Blvd., Suite 1800, Philadelphia, PA 19103-2899. Accounting and Circulation Offices: 6277 Sea Harbor Drive, Orlando, FL 32887-4800. Periodicals postage paid at New York, NY and additional mailing offices. Subscription prices are $125.00 per year (US individuals), $260.00 per year (US institutions), $170.00 per year (Canadian individuals), $340.00 per year (Canadian institutions), $190.00 per year (international individuals), $340.00 per year (international institutions), $65.00 per year (US students), $100.00 per year (Canadian students), and $100.00 per year (foreign students). To receive student/resident rate, orders must be accompanied by name of affiliated institution, date of term, and the signature of program/residency coordinator on institution letterhead. Orders will be billed at individual rate until proof of status is received. Foreign air speed delivery is included in all Clinics subscription prices. All prices are subject to change without notice. POSTMASTER: Send address changes to *The Pediatric Clinics of North America*, Elsevier Periodicals Customer Service, 6277 Sea Harbor Drive, Orlando, FL 32887-4800. **Customer Service: 1-800-654-2452 (US). From outside of the US, call 1-407-345-4000.** E-mail: hhspcs@harcourt.com.

The Pediatric Clinics of North America is also published in Spanish by McGraw-Hill Inter-americana Editores S.A., Mexico City, Mexico; in Portuguese by Reichmann and Affonso Editores, Rua Comandante Coelho 1085, CEP 21250, Rio de Janeiro, Brazil; and in Greek by Althayia SA, Athens, Greece.

The Pediatric Clinics of North America is covered in *Index Medicus, Excerpta Medica, Current Contents, Current Contents/Clinical Medicine, Science Citation Index, ASCA, ISI/BIOMED,* and *BIOSIS.*

Printed in the United States of America.

This book is to be returned on or before
the last date stamped below.

GUEST EDITORS

DONALD VAN WIE, DO, Division of Emergency Medicine, Department of Surgery, Department of Pediatrics; Assistant Program Director, Emergency Medicine/Pediatric Combined Residency Program, University of Maryland School of Medicine, Baltimore, Maryland

GHAZALA Q. SHARIEFF, MD, FACEP, FAAEM, FAAP, Associate Clinical Professor, Children's Hospital and Health Center/University of California; Director, Pediatric Emergency Medicine, Palomar-Pomerado Health System/California Emergency Physicians, San Diego, California

JAMES E. COLLETTI, MD, Assistant Professor of Emergency Medicine, University of Minnesota School of Medicine; Associate Residency Director, Department of Emergency Medicine, Regions Hospital, St. Paul, Minnesota

CONTRIBUTORS

MORGEN BERNIUS, MD, Clinical Instructor, Department of Surgery, Division of Emergency Medicine; EMS Fellow, University of Maryland School of Medicine, Baltimore, Maryland

JAMES E. COLLETTI, MD, Assistant Professor of Emergency Medicine, University of Minnesota School of Medicine; Associate Residency Director, Department of Emergency Medicine, Regions Hospital, St. Paul, Minnesota

LISA DOYLE, MD, Assistant Professor of Clinical Emergency Medicine, Department of Emergency Medicine, University of Arizona University Physicians Hospital, Tucson, Arizona

MARLA J. FRIEDMAN, DO, Attending Physician, Division of Emergency Medicine, Miami Children's Hospital, Miami, Florida

CARSON R. HARRIS, MD, Associate Professor, Department of Emergency Medicine, University of Minnesota Medical School, Minneapolis; Senior Staff, Emergency Medicine Department, Regions Hospital; Director, Clinical Toxicology Service, Emergency Medicine Department, Regions Hospital, St. Paul, Minnesota

KEITH HENRY, MD, Staff Emergency Physician, Emergency Medicine Department, Saint John's Hospital, Maplewood, Minnesota

PAUL ISHIMINE, MD, Assistant Clinical Professor of Medicine and Pediatrics, University of California, San Diego School of Medicine; Director, Pediatric Emergency Medicine, University of California, San Diego Medical Center; Attending Physician, Division of Emergency Medicine, Children's Hospital and Health Center, San Diego, California

RICHARD LICHENSTEIN, MD, Associate Professor, Department of Pediatrics, University of Maryland School of Medicine; Director, Pediatric Emergency Department, University of Maryland Hospital for Children, Baltimore, Maryland

DONNA PERLIN, MD, Assistant Professor of Pediatrics, Division of Pediatric Emergency Medicine, Department of Pediatrics, University of Maryland School of Medicine; Department of Pediatrics, University of Maryland Hospital for Children, Baltimore, Maryland

KEYVAN RAFEI, MD, Assistant Professor, Department of Pediatrics, University of Maryland School of Medicine; Pediatric Emergency Department, University of Maryland Hospital for Children, Baltimore, Maryland

GHAZALA Q. SHARIEFF, MD, FACEP, FAAEM, FAAP, Associate Clinical Professor, Children's Hospital and Health Center/University of California; Director, Pediatric Emergency Medicine, Palomar-Pomerado Health System/California Emergency Physicians, San Diego, California

DONALD VAN WIE, DO, Division of Emergency Medicine, Department of Surgery, Department of Pediatrics; Assistant Program Director, Emergency Medicine/Pediatric Combined Residency Program, University of Maryland School of Medicine, Baltimore, Maryland

STEPHEN WEGNER, MD, Medical Director of Emergency Medical Services; Staff Pediatrician, Blackfeet Community Hospital, Browning, Montana

CONTENTS

department visits and 20% of all pediatric hospital admissions. Causes of upper airway infections include croup, epiglottitis, retropharyngeal abscess, cellulitis, pharyngitis, and peritonsillar abscesses. Lower airway viral and bacterial infections cause illnesses such as pneumonia and bronchiolitis. Signs and symptoms of upper and lower airway infections overlap, but the differentiation is important for appropriate treatment of these conditions. This article reviews the varied clinical characteristics of upper and lower airway infections.

there are several products and medications that are widely available to the pediatric population that can lead to severe toxicity or even death. With some of these medications, death or severe symptoms can occur with the ingestion of only a small amount. It is important that the clinician be familiar with presenting signs and symptoms of potentially toxic ingestions and is able to initiate a therapeutic and life-saving intervention. This article reviews some of the deadlier ingestions that children may be exposed to.

FORTHCOMING ISSUES

RECENT ISSUES

PEDIATRIC CLINICS OF NORTH AMERICA APRIL 2006

GOAL STATEMENT

The goal of *Pediatric Clinics of North America* is to keep practicing physicians and residents up to date with current clinical practice in pediatrics by providing timely articles reviewing the state-of-the-art in patient care.

ACCREDITATION

The *Pediatric Clinics of North America* is planned and implemented in accordance with the Essential Areas and Policies of the Accreditation Council for Continuing Medical Education (ACCME) through the joint sponsorship of the University of Virginia School of Medicine and Elsevier. The University of Virginia School of Medicine is accredited by the ACCME to provide continuing medical education for physicians.

The University of Virginia School of Medicine designates this educational activity for a maximum of 90 category 1 credits per year, 15 category 1 credits per issue, toward the AMA Physician's Recognition Award. Each physician should claim only those credits that he/she actually spent in the activity.

The American Medical Association has determined that physicians not licensed in the US who participate in this CME activity are eligible for 15 AMA PRA Category 1 Credits.

Category 1 credit can be earned by reading the text material, taking the CME examination online at http://www.theclinics.com/home/cme, and completing the evaluation. After taking the test, you will be required to review any and all incorrect answers. Following completion of the test and evaluation, your credit will be awarded and you may print your certificate.

FACULTY DISCLOSURE/CONFLICT OF INTEREST

The University of Virginia School of Medicine, as an ACCME accredited provider, endorses and strives to comply with the Accreditation Council for Continuing Medical Education (ACCME) Standards of Commercial Support, Commonwealth of Virginia statutes, University of Virginia policies and procedures, and associated federal and private regulations and guidelines on the need for disclosure and monitoring of proprietary and financial interests that may affect the scientific integrity and balance of content delivered in continuing medical education activities under our auspices.

The University of Virginia School of Medicine requires that all CME activities accredited through this institution be developed independently and be scientifically rigorous, balanced and objective in the presentation/discussion of its content, theories and practices.

All authors/editors participating in an accredited CME activity are expected to disclose to the readers relevant financial relationships with commercial entities occurring within the past 12 months (such as grants or research support, employee, consultant, stock holder, member of speakers bureau, etc.). The University of Virginia School of Medicine will employ appropriate mechanisms to resolve potential conflicts of interest to maintain the standards of fair and balanced education to the reader. Questions about specific strategies can be directed to the Office of Continuing Medical Education, University of Virginia School of Medicine, Charlottesville, Virginia.

The authors/editors listed below have identified no financial or professional relationships for themselves, their spouse/partner: Morgen J. Bernius, MD; James Colletti, MD; Lisa Doyle, MD; Marla J. Friedman, DO; Carson R. Harris, MD, FAAEM, FACEP; Keith D. Henry, MD; Paul T. Ishimine, MD, FACEP, FAAP; Richard Lichenstein, MD; Donna Perlin, MD; Keyvan Rafei, MD; Ghazala Sharieff, MD; Donald F. Van Wie, Jr., DO; and, Stephen Wegner, MD.

Disclosure of Discussion of Non-FDA Approved Uses for Pharmaceutical and/or Medical Devices: **The University of Virginia School of Medicine, as an ACCME provider, requires that all authors identify and disclose any "off label" uses for pharmaceutical and medical device products. The University of Virginia School of Medicine recommends that each physician fully review all the available data on new products or procedures prior to clinical use.**

TO ENROLL

To enroll in the *Pediatric Clinics of North America* Continuing Medical Education program, call customer service at **1-800-654-2452** or visit us online at www.theclinics.com/home/cme. The CME program is available to subscribers for an additional fee of $195.00.

PEDIATRIC CLINICS

OF NORTH AMERICA

Pediatr Clin N Am 53 (2006) xi–xii

Preface

Pediatric Emergencies, Part II

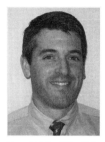
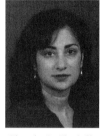
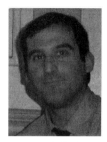

Donald Van Wie, DO

Ghazala Q. Sharieff,
MD, FACEP, FAAEM, FAAP

James E. Colletti, MD

Guest Editors

Children represent our greatest and most vital resource. As such, the need for quality emergency care is an ever-expanding aspect of medicine. Over the last 20 years, significant advances and improvements have occurred in the delivery of emergency care to children, including emergency medicine residency training in pediatric emergencies, pediatric trauma care, pain management for children, pediatric drug dosages, pediatric equipment/supplies in emergency departments and on ambulances, and a national poison control system [1]. Even with these great strides, the practice of pediatric emergency medicine continues to evolve. This issue of *Pediatric Clinics of North America* is the second of two issues this year dedicated to state-of-the-art information regarding the emergency care of children. Current areas of interest, clinical practice, and controversy are addressed.

Exposures to drugs and toxins in the pediatric age group constitute most calls to United States regional poison centers. Several common drugs and toxins can result in potentially deadly ingestions with one or two doses in children. This edition of the *Clinics* discusses several of these deadly ingestions. Procedural sedation and analgesia is a safe, effective, and humane method of managing the pain and anxiety of a child who presents with a painful condition or situation that requires a painful intervention. This issue also discusses an approach to pediatric sedation and analgesia. Fever remains one of the most common chief complaints of children who seek medical attention, and it resulted in more than 5 million

doi:10.1016/j.pcl.2006.02.003
pediatric.theclinics.com

emergency department visits in 2002. Despite the frequency of fever as a chief complaint, considerable controversy remains in the management of this common problem. Current opinions are discussed, including the role vaccinations have played in modifying the approach to young febrile children. The underlying cause of seizures in children may differ from that in adults. Inborn errors of metabolism, child abuse, and immunization reactions can be contributing factors. This issue of the *Clinics* discusses the cause, initial management, and long-term therapy of seizure disorders in children. Despite an increase in awareness and prevention efforts, trauma continues to be one of leading causes of childhood morbidity and mortality. Current concepts in diagnosis and treatment of pediatric blunt abdominal trauma are discussed. To round out this issue, emergent airway infections will be discussed.

We would like to thank all our authors for their time and effort in preparing the manuscripts. We also would like to thank our loving spouses, Jeahan, Arline, and Javaid, and our wonderful children for their support, patience, and understanding during this endeavor.

Donald Van Wie, DO
Office of Emergency Medicine, Department of Surgery and
Department of Pediatrics
University of Maryland School of Medicine
110 S. Paca Street, Sixth Floor, Suite 200
Baltimore, MD 21201, USA
E-mail address: dvanwie@peds.umaryland.edu

Ghazala Q. Sharieff, MD, FACEP, FAAEM, FAAP
Department of Pediatric Emergency Medicine
University of California, San Diego
3030 Children's Way
San Diego, CA 92123, USA
E-mail address: ghazalaqs@hotmail.com

James E. Colletti, MD
Emergency Medicine Regions Hospital
640 Jackson Street
St. Paul, MN 55101-2502, USA
E-mail address: james.e.colletti@healthpartners.com

Reference

[1] American College of Emergency Physicians. A decade of advancements in pediatric emergency care. Available at: www.acep.org/webportal/PatientsConsumers/HealthSubjectsByTopic/Pediatrics/FactSheetADecadeofAdvancementsinPediatricEmergencyCare.htm. Accessed January 31, 2006.

PEDIATRIC CLINICS
OF NORTH AMERICA

ELSEVIER
SAUNDERS

Pediatr Clin N Am 53 (2006) 167–194

Fever Without Source in Children 0 to 36 Months of Age

Paul Ishimine, MD

Department of Emergency Medicine, University of California, San Diego Medical Center,
200 West Arbor Drive, San Diego, CA 92103-8676, USA

Fever, one of the most common chief complaints of children seeking medical attention [1,2], prompted over 5 million emergency department (ED) visits in 2002 [3]. Most of these children have identifiable causes of their fevers, but many will have fever without an apparent source (FWS) after conclusion of the history and physical examination. Despite the frequency of fever as a chief complaint, there is considerable controversy in the management of the young child who has FWS [4–8]. The challenge in the evaluation of the febrile young child lies in balancing the minimization of risk to the patient with the costs of testing and treatment.

Definition of fever

A variety of temperatures have been used to define fever, but the most commonly accepted definition of fever is a temperature of $\geq 38.0°C$ (100.4°F), a value derived from studies by Wunderlich, who took 1 million measurements on 25,000 patients and determined that this temperature was the upper limit of normal [9]. Although less invasive means of measuring temperature exist, such as axillary and aural thermometry, the variability of measurements at these sites [10–12] warrants using the current outpatient reference standard, rectal thermometry, when measuring temperatures in young children. An accurate temperature measurement is especially important if a practitioner chooses to use fever guidelines because the implementation of these guidelines is initiated once a patient meets a certain temperature threshold.

E-mail address: pishimin@ucsd.edu

Once it is determined that a child has a fever, measured in the emergency department or in the practitioner's office, further evaluation can then proceed. However, a child who presents with a reported fever at home but who is afebrile in the ED or in the office poses more of a challenge. Parents may not be able to accurately define fever [13], and subjective assessment by parents has been shown to have generally good but variable sensitivity in the detection of fever [14–16]. Parental assessment is often colored by "fever phobia," inaccurate concerns and misconceptions about the potential danger of fever [17,18]. Additionally, bundling of infant creates confusion for both providers and parents because bundling of infants may raise the skin temperature but not rectal temperature [19]. However, a fever measured at home with rectal thermometry generally warrants the same concern as a fever measured in the ED or in the office. Six of 63 patients with bacteremia or bacterial meningitis in a large office-based study of young febrile infants were found to be afebrile in physicians' offices but were febrile at home [20].

Epidemiology

The management of the febrile young child continues to evolve. Contributing to this confusion is the changing epidemiology of bacterial infection in young children. *Haemophilus influenzae* previously presented a significant burden of disease, resulting in substantial morbidity and mortality in young children. *H influenzae* represented 19% of all positive cultures in febrile children who presented to a pediatric walk-in clinic in 1972 [21], but after widespread use of the *H influenzae* type b vaccine starting in 1991, the epidemiology of invasive bacterial disease changed dramatically. *H influenzae* type b has been nearly eliminated [22,23], with a 94% decline in *H influenzae* meningitis shortly after the introduction of the Hib vaccine [24]. Combining the results of two large studies of occult bacteremia in patients seen in the mid 1990s in Boston and Philadelphia, there were no blood cultures that grew *H influenzae* from 15,366 patients seen in these pediatric emergency departments [25,26].

Corresponding to the decrease in invasive disease caused by *H influenzae*, there has been an increase in the percentage of invasive diseases caused by *Streptococcus pneumoniae*. The burden of disease caused by *S pneumoniae* has been significant. *S pneumoniae* represented 83% to 92% of positive blood cultures taken from young febrile children presenting to EDs in the mid 1990s, and the overall prevalence of occult bacteremia was 1.6% to 1.9% [25,26]. In 1998, there were an estimated 12,560 cases of invasive pneumococcal disease (bacteremia, meningitis, and pneumonia) and 110 deaths in children younger than 2 years of age, with a case fatality rate of 1.4% [27]. This low overall case fatality rate likely reflects the generally good outcomes in patients with bacteremia, which represented 75% of the invasive disease in this population [27]. However, the case fatality rate resulting from *S pneumoniae* meningitis is higher than meningitis caused by *Neisseria meningitidis*, *Streptococcus* group B, *Listeria monocytogenes*, or *H influenzae* [24]. Additionally, there has been an increasing prevalence of multidrug resistant *S pneumoniae*, and the proportion of isolates with multidrug resistance is highest in children under 5 years of age [28,29]. Although an effective, 23-valent polysaccharide pneumococcal vaccine has been licensed since 1983, this vaccine is insufficiently immunogenic in young children and is, therefore, ineffective and not recommended for children younger than 2 years of age, which is the age group most at risk for invasive pneumococcal infection.

The introduction of the heptavalent pneumococcal conjugate vaccine (PCV7), covering the seven most common pneumococcal serotypes, has changed the landscape of invasive bacterial disease in young children. There are over 90 pneumococcal serotypes that have been identified, but the seven serotypes included in the vaccine (4, 6B, 9V, 14, 18C, 19F, and 23F) cause approximately 82% of the cases of invasive pneumococcal disease [27]. This vaccine, licensed in 2000, is recommended for universal administration to children younger than 2 years old in a 4-dose regimen (doses are given at 2, 4, 6, and 12–15 months), as well as to high-risk older children (eg, children with sickle cell disease, chronic cardiac and pulmonary diseases, and other immunocompromising conditions) [30].

This vaccine has been shown to be both safe [31] and highly effective in preventing invasive pneumococcal disease, with a prelicensure study demonstrating an efficacy of 97% [32]. In a postlicensure surveillance of the Northern California Kaiser Permanente [32] study cohort, the cohort that served as the largest prelicensure study group of the PCV7 vaccine, the incidence of invasive pneumococcal disease caused by vaccine and cross-reactive vaccine serotypes declined from 51.5 to 98.2 cases of invasive disease per 100,000 person-years in children less than 1 year old to 0 cases per 100,000 person-years 4 years after licensure [33]. There was also a reduction of invasive pneumococcal disease in children less than 2 years old, declining from 81.7 to 113.8 cases of invasive disease per 100,000 person-years to 0 cases per 100,000 person-years 4 years after the vaccine was licensed [33]. There was a decline in invasive pneumococcal disease for all serotypes, not just the seven covered by PCV7, with a decline of 94% and 91% in children less than 1 year of age and 2 years of age, respectively. There was also a significant decline in drug-resistant pneumococci and a 25% decrease in invasive pneumococcal disease in people older than 5 years old, suggesting herd immunity because these patients were not themselves immunized. These declines occurred despite the fact that only 24% of children less than 2 years old received all four recommended doses because of a vaccine shortage [33].

These findings have been replicated in other settings. In Massachusetts, there was a 69% decline in the incidence of total invasive pneumococcal disease as well as an 88% decline in non-meningitis vaccine-serotype disease [34]. Similarly, there was a 69% decline in the total incidence of invasive pneumococcal disease and a 78% decline in the incidence of disease caused by vaccine serotypes, seen in a national network of regional surveillance centers administered by the Centers for Disease Control and Prevention, accompanied by a decline in penicillin-resistant pneumococcal isolates [35]. There was a 66% decline in the incidence of invasive pneumococcal infections (77% decline in vaccine-covered serotypes) noted from a network study of children's hospitals [36]. Three likely mechanisms are involved in the PCV7-associated decrease in disease: individual risk decline, decline in antibiotic-resistant bacteria, and herd immunity.

Caveats

Although the differential diagnosis of fever is quite broad and includes both infectious and noninfectious causes [37], the majority of febrile children have underlying infectious causes of fever. For the purposes of this article, patients are presumed to be febrile from infectious sources. Additionally, diagnostic strategies emphasize the detection of bacterial disease because bacterial diseases are more likely to be associated with worse outcomes, but viral infections can also be associated with significant morbidity and mortality, especially in younger children.

Most large studies addressing serious bacterial illness use children from large, urban, tertiary care children's hospital emergency departments. Physicians in primary care settings are less compliant with ED-derived recommendations for the evaluation and treatment of febrile children, but compared with ED patients, outcomes for these patients are similar [20,38]. This similarity in outcome may be the result of several causes: the sickest patients may preferentially present to the ED, patients may get closer follow-up by their primary care providers, the judgment of primary care providers may be more sensitive than criteria put forth in various guidelines, or because the likelihood of serious disease in these children is low [39].

Finally, most studies of febrile young children exclude patients who have potentially complicating risk factors. These studies typically have excluded children who are immunocompromised (eg, sickle cell disease, cancer, or long-term steroid use), have indwelling medical devices (eg, ventriculoperitoneal shunts and indwelling venous access catheters), are currently taking antibiotics, or have prolonged fevers (≥ 5 days).

Approach to the young febrile child

History and physical examination

The history and physical examination are invaluable in the assessment of the febrile child. The level and duration of a child's fever as well as the mode of temperature measurement are important to note. There is an increase in the prevalence of pneumococcal bacteremia with an increase in temperature [40], and this is more pronounced in young children. In children less than 3 months of age who have temperatures $\geq 40.0°C$, 38% have serious bacterial infection [41]. The duration of the fever itself at the time of ED presentation does not predict whether a child has occult bacteremia [42]. The use of antipyretics should be noted. Parents often give inaccurate doses of antipyretics [43,44], and paradoxically, in one study, patients treated with antipyretics presented to the ED with higher temperatures than those patients who were untreated at home [45]. A response (or lack thereof) to antipyretic medications does not predict whether the underlying cause is bacterial or viral [45–49]. Additional important data include associated signs and symptoms, underlying medical conditions, exposure to ill contacts, and immunization status.

An assessment of the child's overall appearance is critical. If a child appears to be toxic, this mandates an aggressive work-up, antibiotic treatment, and hospitalization, regardless of age or risk factors. The physical examination may reveal obvious sources of infection, and the identification of a focal infection may decrease the need for additional testing. For example, febrile patients with recognizable viral conditions (eg, croup, chickenpox, and stomatitis) have lower rates of bacteremia than patients with no obvious source of infection [50]. Similarly, febrile children with influenzavirus A have lower rates of serious bacterial infections compared with febrile children without influenzavirus A [51]. Febrile patients with otitis media appear to have the same rate of bacteremia as febrile children without otitis media [52,53].

With the exception of neonates and young infants, if a child has a nontoxic appearance, a more selective approach can be undertaken. When a child who has a febrile illness has an obviously identifiable cause, the treatment and disposition should generally be tailored to this specific infection. The approach to the young child who has FWS is discussed below.

Age-specific considerations

The approach to the young child who has a fever without a source varies depending on the age of the child. Traditionally, young children have been categorized in into three distinct age groups for the purposes of fever evaluation: the neonate (0–28 days old), the young infant (commonly defined as infants between 1 and 3 months of age, although some authors define this group to include children only between 1 and 2 months of age), and the older infant or toddler (commonly defined as 3 to 36 months of age, although some studies include patients only up to 24 months old in this group). Although the use of chronologic age distinctions are somewhat artificial (for example, the difference in the risk of serious bacterial illness is likely to be inconsequentially different between a 28-day-old child and a 29-day-old child), there is some rationale behind these seemingly arbitrary age distinctions. Younger children have decreased immunologic function and are more commonly infected with virulent organisms. Additionally, the physical examination is more difficult because young children have a limited behavioral repertoire.

Young infants: 0 to 3 months old

The traditional approach to young infants has included aggressive investigation, antibiotic administration, and hospital admission [54]. However, the hospitalization of young infants can result in iatrogenic complications, financial ramifications, and parental stress [55,56]. Recently, this approach has been challenged, and the current recommendations are not as strict regarding mandatory admission in well-appearing infants over 28 days old.

Neonates: birth to 28 days old

Neonates are at a particularly high risk for SBI. The majority of febrile neonates presenting to the ED are diagnosed ultimately as having a nonspecific viral illness, but approximately 12% of all febrile neonates presenting to a pediatric emergency department have serious bacterial illness [57,58]. When they are infected, neonates are infected typically by more virulent bacteria (eg, *Streptococci* group B, *Escherichia coli*, and *L monocytogenes*) and are more likely to develop serious sequelae from viral infections (eg, herpes simplex virus meningitis). *Streptococci* group B, a common bacteria pathogen in this age group, is associated with high rates of meningitis (39%), non-meningeal foci of infection (10%), and sepsis (7%) [59]. This age group is the least likely to be affected by the use of the pneumococcal vaccine because only a small percentage of neonates are infected by this pathogen. Although infection is uncommon, those neonates who are infected with *S pneumonia* have a mortality rate of 14% [60]. The most common bacterial infections in this are group are urinary tract infections (UTIs) and occult bacteremia [57,58].

Evaluation of the febrile neonate

Traditional risk-stratification strategies have used ancillary testing to supplement the limited information available from the history and physical examination. Unfortunately, it is difficult to predict accurately which neonates have invasive disease, even when laboratory testing is used. Initial studies by Dagan and colleagues [61,62] appeared promising. These "Rochester criteria" (Rochester, Boston, and Philadelphia criteria are discussed below) were applied to infants less than 90 days old, and neonates were included. Using the Rochester criteria, Jaskiewicz and colleagues [63] found that 2 of 227 children younger than 30 days old who met low-risk criteria had SBI. However, Ferrera and colleagues [64] found that 6% of neonates who were retrospectively classified as low risk by the Rochester criteria had SBI.

Baker and colleagues [65] retrospectively stratified neonates into high- and low-risk patients based on the "Philadelphia criteria" they had derived for older infants. The neonates who were placed in the high-risk category had a higher incidence of bacterial disease (18.6%), but 4.6% of neonates who were classified as low-risk patients had a serious bacterial infection. Additionally, 11 different bacterial pathogens were identified in 32 patients with SBI, and only one of these 32 patients was infected with *S pneumoniae*. Kadish and colleagues [58] found a similar rate of SBI in neonates whom they categorized as low risk when they retrospectively applied both the Philadelphia criteria and similar criteria created by Baskin and colleagues (the "Boston criteria"). They also found a wide range of bacterial pathogens, but only two cultures in 55 patients with SBI were positive from *S pneumoniae*.

Because of the inability to accurately predict serious infections in this age group, the recommendations for these patients include obtaining blood cultures, urine for rapid urine testing, urine cultures, and cerebrospinal fluid (CSF) [66,67]. A peripheral white blood cell (WBC) count is often ordered in the evaluation of febrile neonates, but the discriminatory value of the WBC count is insufficient to differentiate between patients with SBI versus nonbacterial infection [68–70]. Because of the inability of the white blood cell count to predict SBI, blood cultures should be ordered on all patients. Although various options for rapidly testing for urinary tract infection exist (eg, urine dipstick, standard urinalysis, and enhanced urinalysis), no rapid test detects all cases of UTI, so urine cultures must be ordered in all of these patients [71,72]. Urine should be collected by bladder catheterization or suprapubic aspiration because bag urine specimens are associated with unacceptably high rates of contamination [73,74]. A lumbar puncture should be performed in all febrile neonates. Chest radiographs are indicated only in the presence of respiratory symptoms, and stool analyses are indicated only in the presence of diarrhea. In neonates, the presence of signs suggestive of viral illness does not negate the need for a full diagnostic evaluation. Unlike older children, in whom documented respiratory syncytial virus (RSV) infections decrease the likelihood of serious bacterial illness, RSV-infected neonates have the same rate of SBI compared with RSV-negative neonates [75].

Treatment and disposition of the febrile neonate

Because of the high rates of serious bacterial infections, all febrile neonates should receive antibiotics. Typically, these patients are treated with a third-generation cephalosporin or gentamicin. Ceftriaxone is not recommended for neonates who have jaundice because of the concern for inducing unconjugated hyperbilirubinemia [76–78]. Other third-generation cephalosporins, such as cefotaxime, 50 mg/kg intravenously (IV) (100 mg/kg if there is a concern for meningitis based on CSF results), or gentamicin, 2.5 mg/kg IV, are used in this age group. Additionally, although the incidence of *L monocytogenes* is quite low [79], ampicillin, 50 mg/kg IV (100 mg/kg IV if there is a concern for meningitis) is still recommended in the empiric treatment of these patients [80].

Neonatal herpes simplex virus (HSV) infections occur in approximately 1 per 3200 deliveries in the United States [81]. Neonates with HSV infections usually present within the first 2 weeks of life, and only a minority of infected children have fever [82]. Rates of morbidity and mortality are high with neonatal HSV, but treatment with high-dose acyclovir improves outcomes in patients [83]. Acyclovir is not recommended routinely for empiric treatment in addition to standard antibiotics in febrile neonates [82] but should be considered in febrile neonates with risk factors for neonatal HSV (20 mg/kg IV). Risk factors include primary maternal infection, especially those neonates delivered vaginally, prolonged rupture of membranes at delivery, the use of fetal scalp electrodes, skin, eye or mouth lesions, seizures, and CSF pleocytosis [81,84,85].

Febrile neonates should be hospitalized, regardless of the results of laboratory studies. Outpatient management of these patients has been suggested [86] and occurs frequently when patients present to pediatricians' offices [20]. However, given the lack of prospective studies addressing this approach as well as the limitations inherent in the screening evaluation in the emergency department and frequent difficulties in arranging follow-up evaluation, hospitalization is strongly recommended [66,67].

Young infants: 1 to 3 months old

The approach to febrile young infants, defined most commonly as children less than either 2 or 3 months old (in this discussion, age less than 3 months will be used), changed dramatically in the 1980s and early 1990s. Before this time, most febrile young infants presenting to academic medical centers were hospitalized and frequently started on antibiotic therapy. The aggressive approach was based in part on the relatively limited amount of information obtainable from examination of young infants [65,87], the high morbidity rate observed with *H influenzae* type b infection, and the efficacy of antibiotics in the treatment of serious bacterial infection.

The "Rochester criteria" put forth by Dagan and colleagues [61,62] stratified children less than 60 days old into high- and low-risk groups. The children who met these criteria appeared well, had been previously healthy, and had no evidence of skin, soft tissue, bone, joint, or ear infection. Additionally, the children had normal peripheral WBC count ($5000–15,000/mm^3$), normal absolute band counts ($\leq 1500/mm^3$), ≤ 10 WBC/high-power field (hpf) of centrifuged urine sediment, and for those patients with diarrhea, ≤ 5 WBC/hpf on stool smear [61,62]. The low-risk group identified children who were unlikely to have serious bacterial infection, with a negative predictive value of 98.9% [63].

In 1992, Baskin and colleagues [88] described the "Boston criteria" for febrile children between 1 and 3 months of age who presented to the emergency department with temperatures $\geq 38.0°C$. Infants were discharged after an intramuscular (IM) injection ceftriaxone, 50 mg/kg, if they generally appeared to be well (not strictly defined) and had no ear, soft tissue, joint, or bone infections on physical examination. Furthermore, these patients had to have CSF with ≤ 10 WBC/hpf, microscopic UA with ≤ 10 WBC/hpf or urine dipstick negative for leukocyte esterase, a peripheral WBC count of $\leq 20,000/mm^3$, and normal findings in patients in whom a chest radiograph was obtained (all tests except the chest radiograph were performed on all patients). Twenty-seven of

503 children (5.4%) were later found to have serious bacterial infection (bacterial gastroenteritis, urinary tract infection, and occult bacteremia). Only one of nine patients with occult bacteremia in this study were infected *S pneumoniae* [88].

Baker and colleagues [65] similarly sought to identify low-risk patients between 29 and 56 days old with temperatures of $\geq 38.2°C$. Patients who appeared to be well (as defined by an Infant Observation Score of 10 or less), had a peripheral WBC count of $\leq 15,000/mm^3$, a band-to-neutrophil ratio of ≤ 0.2, a urinalysis (UA) with fewer than 10 WBC/hpf, few or no bacteria on a centrifuged urine specimen, CSF with fewer than 8 WBC/mm^3, a gram-negative stain, negative results on chest radiographs (obtained on all patients), and stool negative for blood and few or no WBCs on microscopy (ordered on those patients with watery diarrhea) were considered to have a negative screen and were not treated with antibiotics. Of the 747 consecutively enrolled patients, 65 (8.7%) had SBI. All 65 patients who had serious bacterial infection were identified using these screening criteria. These 65 patients had a total of 70 bacterial infection sites where a bacterial pathogen was identified, and four of these 70 infections were caused by *S pneumoniae* [65]. In a follow-up study (in which fever was defined as $\geq 38.0°C$ rectally) of 422 consecutively enrolled febrile young infants, 43 (10%) had SBI, and all 101 patients who were identified as low risk had no SBI. All 43 patients who had SBI were identified prospectively as high risk using the Philadelphia criteria [89].

In the large studies by Baskin and Baker and colleagues, only a minority of patients with SBI had pneumococcal infection, and thus, children in this age group are unlikely to benefit directly from the PCV7 vaccine [65,88].

Evaluation of the febrile young infant

The clinical evaluation alone will result in a substantial number of missed SBI, so laboratory testing is required in this age group. The white blood cell count with differential, catheterized urinalysis, and blood and urine cultures should be obtained in all patients. Stool studies for white blood cell counts and stool cultures should be ordered in patients with diarrhea. Chest radiographs should be obtained only in young febrile infants with signs of pulmonary disease (tachypnea ≥ 50 breaths/minute, rales, rhonchi, retractions, wheezing, coryza, grunting, nasal flaring, or cough) [90,91].

Controversies in this age group surround the need for lumbar puncture. Although the Boston and Philadelphia criteria require CSF analysis, the Rochester criteria do not mandate lumbar puncture. The rarity of bacterial meningitis contributes to the controversy surrounding the utility of the lumbar puncture. However, the prevalence of bacterial meningitis in febrile infants less than 3 months old is 4.1 per 1000 patients, and neither the clinical examination nor the peripheral white blood cell count is reliable in diagnosing meningitis in this age group [68,92]; therefore, the LP should be strongly considered. Additional controversy surrounds the need for antibiotics in patients who are identified as low risk. Patients identified as low risk by the Philadelphia protocol were not given antibiotics, whereas patients enrolled in the Boston studies were given intramuscular ceftriaxone. There is some concern that performing a lumbar puncture in a bacteremic patient may lead to meningitis [93,94], and published recommendations state that parenteral antibiotics should be "considered" if a lumbar puncture is performed [66].

The results of these tests help to risk-stratify these young children. The WBC count is considered abnormal if the count is $\geq 15{,}000/mm^3$ or $\leq 5000/mm^3$ and the band- to-neutrophil ratio is ≥ 0.2. The urine is considered abnormal if the urine dipstick is positive for nitrite or leukocyte esterase; or there are ≥ 5 WBC/hpf on microscopy; or organisms are seen on a Gram-stained sample of un-centrifuged urine. If obtained, there should be fewer than 5 WBC/hpf on the stool specimen, no evidence of pneumonia on chest x-ray, and fewer than 8 WBC/mm^3 and no organisms on Gram stain of the cerebrospinal fluid [66]. Of note, however, one recent study reported that four of 8300 children who underwent CSF analysis had bacterial meningitis and ≤ 8 WBC/mm^3 in the CSF [95].

The presence of a documented viral infection lowers but does not eliminate the likelihood of a serious bacterial infection in this age group. Young infants classified as high-risk patients using the Rochester criteria who had documented viral infection (enterovirus, respiratory virus, rotavirus, and herpesvirus) were at lower risk for SBI compared with patients who did not have an identified source (4.2% versus 12.3%) [96]. Similarly, a subgroup analysis of 187 febrile infants 28 to 60 days old showed a significantly lower rate of SBI in RSV-positive patients compared with RSV-negative patients (5.5% versus 11.7%) [75], confirming the results of similar studies in young infants who had bronchiolitis. Most of these bacterial infections were urinary tract infections [97,98]. Patients less than 90 days old who have enteroviral infections have a rate of concurrent serious bacterial infections (mostly UTI) of 7% [99].

Treatment and disposition of the febrile young infant

Assuming that the patient is an otherwise healthy term infant who appears to be well and who does not have any lab abnormalities, outpatient management may be considered. If the patient undergoes a reliable follow-up within 24 hours, the parents have a way of immediately accessing health care if there is a change in the patient's condition, and the parents and the primary care physician understand and agree with this plan of care, then the patient may be discharged home. The use of ceftriaxone, 50 mg/kg IV or IM, before discharge is acceptable, as is withholding antibiotics in these low-risk patients. Patients who did not undergo lumbar puncture in the ED should not receive antibiotics because this will confound the evaluation for meningitis if the patient is still febrile on follow-up examination. Close follow-up reevaluation must be assured before discharge.

For those patients who have abnormal test results or who appear to be ill, antibiotic therapy and hospitalization are warranted. Ceftriaxone, 50 mg/kg IM or IV (100 mg/kg if meningitis is suspected), is commonly used for these patients.

Additional antibiotics should be considered in select circumstances (eg, ampicillin or vancomycin for suspected infection by *Listeria*, gram-positive cocci, or enterococcus). Some studies suggest that patients in this age group who have urinary tract infections may be treated on an outpatient basis [100,101]; however, there are no prospective studies with a large number of young infants that address this question.

Older infants and toddlers: 3 to 36 months old

A temperature of $\geq 38.0°C$ defines a fever, and in younger children, this temperature is the usual threshold beyond which diagnostic testing is initiated. However, in febrile children between 3 and 36 months old (some studies extend this group to include 2-month-old infants), a temperature of $\geq 39.0°C$ is commonly used as the threshold temperature for initiating further evaluation. This higher temperature cutoff is used because of the increasing risk of occult bacteremia with increasing temperatures [40]. Large studies of occult bacteremia, widely referenced in the medical literature, use this temperature as the study entry criteria [25,26,102].

Evaluation of the child 3 to 36 months old

The history is often helpful in this age group. Patients are more likely to be able to communicate complaints, and the physical examination is more informative. Clinical assessment as to whether a child appears to be well, ill, or toxic is important. A well appearance does not completely exclude bacteremia [103], but children who appear toxic are much more likely to have serious illness compared with ill- or well-appearing children (92% versus 26% versus 3%, respectively) [104]. Many bacterial infections can be identified by history and physical examination alone, but some infections may be occult. The serious bacterial infections that may not be clinically apparent are bacteremia, urinary tract infection, and pneumonia. If no focal source of infection is identified and the cause is not believed to be viral, then diagnostic testing in this age group is undertaken for the purposes of identifying these occult bacterial infections.

Occult bacteremia

In the era before universal PCV7 vaccination, the pathogen that most commonly caused occult bacteremia was *S pneumoniae* [25,26]. The children at greatest risk for pneumococcal bacteremia are children between 6 and 24 months old. There has been much controversy about the role of blood testing in the evaluation of the febrile child, specifically regarding the value of blood testing in the identification of occult bacteremia. There is an increased risk of bacteremia with an increasing white blood cell count [26,105,106], but the sensitivity and specificity of a white blood cell count $\geq 15,000/mm^3$ is only 80% to 86% and 69% to 77%, respectively. An absolute neutrophil count (ANC) of $\geq 10,000/mm^3$ is a stronger predictor of occult bacteremia than an elevated white blood cell count. Eight percent of patients who have an ANC $\geq 10,000/mm$ have occult pneumococcal bacteremia, whereas 0.8% of patients who have an ANC $\leq 10,000/mm^3$ have occult pneumococcal bacteremia [40]. Nevertheless, using an elevated WBC or ANC as a surrogate marker for occult bacteremia means that many patients will unnecessarily receive antibiotics.

The shifting epidemiology of bacteremia has prompted cost-effectiveness analyses of various management strategies. Using pre-PCV7 data, Lee and colleagues [107] analyzed five strategies for the 3- to 36-month-old febrile child who did not have an identifiable source of infection. Using a bacteremia prevalence rate of 1.5%, the authors concluded that the most cost-efficient strategy was to obtain CBCs and to selectively send blood cultures and treat patients empirically for WBC counts $>15,000/mm^3$. In their sensitivity analysis, the authors found that when the prevalence rate of pneumococcal bacteremia dropped to 0.5%, then clinical judgment (eg, the patient who was deemed to be at low risk clinically for occult pneumococcal bacteremia received no testing) was a more cost-effective strategy.

The role of antibiotics in children believed to be at high-risk for bacteremia is controversial as well. There is currently no way of prospectively identifying bacteremic patients, and practically, this means that at the time of the ED or office visit, many febrile children who are at risk for bacteremia must be treated to prevent a single serious bacterial infection. The use of both amoxicillin [108] and ceftriaxone [102,105] appears to shorten the duration of fever in bacteremic febrile children. However, there is a paucity of randomized, placebo-controlled data demonstrating that the use of either oral or parenteral antibiotics prevents significant, adverse infectious sequelae in these children. One study compared amoxicillin with placebo for the treatment of febrile children and showed no difference in the rates of subsequent focal infection [108]. Another retrospective study demonstrated that, in patients ultimately found to have bacteremia, treatment with oral or parenteral antibiotics reduced persistent fever, persistent bacteremia, and hospital admission [109]. A subsequent meta-analysis has shown that, although ceftriaxone prevents serious bacterial infection in patients with proven occult bacteremia, 284 patients at risk for bacteremia would need to be treated with antibiotics to prevent one case of meningitis [110]. Although oral antibiotics also decrease the risk of SBI in patients with occult bacteremia caused by S pneumoniae, it is unclear whether antibiotics reduce the risk of meningitis in these patients [111]. Additionally, there is no apparent difference in rates of serious bacterial infection in patients with occult pneumococcal bacteremia who are treated with oral versus parenteral antibiotics [112]. Complicating this analysis is the fact that in a majority of patients with pneumococcal bacteremia, the bacteremia will resolve spontaneously [25]. Focal infections develop in 17% of bacteremic children [25], and 2.7% to 5.8% of patients with occult pneumococcal bacteremia develop meningitis [111,113]. These analyses were conducted on data obtained in the pre-PCV7 era, and it is likely, with the significant decrease in invasive pneumococcal disease, that many more febrile patients will need to be treated to prevent SBI.

There are relatively few data on occult bacteremia in the post-PCV7 era. In one retrospective cohort study of pediatric emergency department patients, three of 329 blood cultures in children between 2 to 36 months old were positive for S pneumoniae. One patient was infected with a nonvaccine serotype, one was not immunized with PCV7, and a third patient was infected with an unknown serotype [114].

Although pneumococcus has been the most common cause of occult bacteremia, other causes of bacteremia can be occult as well. Salmonella causes 4% of occult bacteremia, occurring in 0.1% of all children 3 to 36 months old who have temperatures $\geq 39.0°C$ [25,26,102], and whereas the majority of patients with Salmonella bacteremia have gastroenteritis, 5% will have primary bacteremia [115]. One large retrospective study of non-typhi Salmonella bacteremia in children showed that 54% of bacteremic children had a temperature $\leq 39.0°C$ and a median WBC count of $10,000/mm^3$. These children had a 41% rate of persistent bacteremia on follow-up cultures, and the rates of persistent bacteremia were the same in patients who were treated with antibiotics at the initial visit and those who were not. Among immunocompetent patients, 2.5% of patients with Salmonella bacteremia had focal infections, and no difference in rates of focal infection were noted in children older and younger than 3 months of age [116].

Meningococcal infections are infrequent causes of bacteremia but are associated with high rates of morbidity and mortality. Combining the data from Boston and Philadelphia occult bacteremia studies, 0.02% of children who appeared to be nontoxic and had temperatures $\geq 39.0°C$ had meningococcal disease [25,26]. Usually, these patients are overtly sick; however, 12% to 16% of patients with meningococcal disease have unsuspected infection [117,118]. Although there is an association between younger age and elevated band count with meningococcal disease, the positive predictive values of these variables are quite low, given the low prevalence of this disease, and authors of one large meningococcal disease study believe that routine screening for all young febrile children with CBCs for meningococcal bacteremia is not useful [117]. Patients who had unsuspected meningococcal disease who were treated empirically with antibiotics had fewer complications than patients who were untreated, but there were no differences in rates of permanent sequelae or death [119]. However, testing and empiric treatment may be warranted for children at higher risk for meningococcal disease. Risk factors for meningoccal bacteremia include contact with patients with meningoccal disease, periods of meningoccal disease outbreaks, and presence of fever and petechiae (although the majority of children with fever and petechiae do not have invasive bacterial disease) [120–122]. A new tetravalent meningococcal conjugate vaccine was licensed for use in the United States in 2005. Although clinical trials in infants and young children are in

progress, this vaccine has been licensed and recommended for routine administration only in children 11 years old and older [123].

Children who have positive blood cultures need to be reexamined. A patient
who appears ill needs a repeat blood culture, lumbar puncture, intravenous
antibiotics, and hospital admission. Patients with pneumococcal bacteremia who
are afebrile on repeat evaluation can be followed on an outpatient basis [124]
after repeated blood cultures and antibiotics. Children who have pneumococcal
bacteremia and who are persistently febrile need repeat blood cultures and
generally should undergo lumbar puncture and require hospital admission. The
treatment and disposition for well-appearing children with *Salmonella* bacteremia
are less clear, but patients with meningococcal bacteremia should be hospitalized
for parenteral antibiotics [106].

Contaminated blood cultures are common, and in younger children, the rate
of contaminated cultures frequently exceeds the rate of true positive cultures
[25,26,114,125,126]. Although the average cost to the patient of a false-positive
blood culture is rather small [127], false-positive blood cultures lead to further
testing, use of antibiotics, and hospitalizations [128], along with the attendant
iatrogenic complications [129]. The rates of blood culture contamination decline
when cultures are drawn from a separate site rather than through a newly inserted
intravenous catheter [126].

Given the observed decline in invasive pneumococcal disease, the relative
infrequency of meningococcemia and *Salmonella* bacteremia, and the limited
value of the white blood cell count in predicting the latter two diseases, the need
for routine CBC, blood cultures, and empiric antibiotics have been called into
question in fully immunized children [130,131]. Baraff, the author of the commonly referenced fever algorithms [66,132], has recently stated that children
who have received three does of vaccine are at sufficiently low risk that they do
not need blood testing or antibiotics and that patients who have received only two
doses of the Hib and PCV7 vaccines are not at any significant risk for occult
bacteremia [133]. It is reasonable to address parental preferences when devising a
"risk-minimizing" versus a "test-minimizing" [134] approach to these children
because parental perceptions and preferences regarding risk may differ from
those of the treating clinician.

Occult urinary tract infection

UTIs are common sources of fever in young children, and children are at risk
for permanent renal damage from UTIs. In older children, historical and examination features such as dysuria, urinary frequency, and abdominal and flank
pain may suggest urinary tract infection. However, in young children, symptoms
are usually nonspecific. Although the overall prevalence in children is 2% to 5%
[135–137], certain subgroups of children are at higher risk for UTIs. Whites,
girls, uncircumcised boys, no alternative source of fever, and temperatures
≥ 39.0°C were associated with a higher risk; 16% of white girls less than 2 years

old with temperatures $\geq 39.0^\circ$C and fever without source had urinary tract infections [135,136]. UTIs were found in 2.7% to 3.5% of febrile children, even when there were other potential sources of fever (eg, gastroenteritis, otitis media, upper respiratory tract infection, and nonspecific rash) [135,136].

Based on these prevalence data, a clinical decision rule was derived and validated for febrile girls less than 24 months of age. Urine testing is indicated if two or more of the following risk factors are present: age less than 12 months, fever for 2 or more days, temperature $\geq 39.0^\circ$C, white, and no alternative source of fever [138]. This rule has a sensitivity of 95% to 99% and a false-positive rate 69% to 90% in detecting girls with UTI [138,139]. No similar clinical decision rules exist for boys, but because the prevalence in boys less than 6 months old is 2.7% [136], urine should be collected in all boys in this age group. The prevalence of UTIs in uncircumcised boys is 8 to 9 times higher than circumcised boys, so uncircumcised boys younger than 12 months old should also undergo urine testing [136,140,141].

Urine culture is the gold standard for the diagnosis of urinary tract infection, but results are not immediately available. Several rapid urine tests have very good sensitivity for detecting UTIs. Enhanced urinalysis (≥ 10 WBC/hpf or bacteria on Gram stained, uncentrifuged urine) [71,142] or a combination of ≥ 10 WBC/hpf and bacteriuria (on either centrifuged or uncentrifuged urine) [143] are both excellent screening tests. The more readily available urine dipstick (positive for either leukocyte esterase or nitrites) has a sensitivity of 88% [71]. Importantly, however, because no rapid screening test detected all UTIs, urine cultures should be ordered on all of these patients [74]. Any positive test results from a rapid test should lead to a presumptive diagnosis of a urinary tract infection, and antibiotic treatment should be initiated. Most patients with urinary tract infection who appear well can be treated on an outpatient basis. Empiric antibiotic therapy should be tailored to local bacterial epidemiology, but reasonable outpatient medications include cefixime (8 mg/kg twice on the first day of treatment, then 8 mg/kg/d, starting from the second day) or cephalexin (25–100 mg/kg/d divided into four doses). The duration of therapy should be from 7 to 14 days.

Occult pneumonia

Young children commonly develop pneumonia, and the most common pathogens are viruses and (based on pre-PCV7 data) *S pneumoniae* [144]. The diagnosis of pneumonia based on clinical examination can be difficult [145]. Multiple attempts have been made at deriving clinical decision rules for the accurate diagnosis of pneumonia, but none has been successfully validated [146–148]. The presence of any pulmonary findings on examination (eg, tachypnea, crackles, respiratory distress, or decreased breath sounds) increases the likelihood of pneumonia, and conversely, the absence of these findings decreases the likelihood of pneumonia [149–151]. The role of pulse oximetry in detecting pneumonia is unclear [152,153], and although the chest radiograph is often believed to be the gold standard, there is variability in the interpretation of radiographs even by pediatric radiologists [154]. Radiographic findings cannot be used to distinguish reliably between bacterial and nonbacterial causes [155,156]. In one South African study, chest radiographs did not affect the clinical outcome in children meeting the World Health Organization definition of pneumonia [157].

Some cases of pneumonia are likely to be clinically occult. Bachur and colleagues [158] found that 19% to 26% of children younger than 5 years old who had a temperature of $\geq 39.0°C$, a WBC count $\geq 20,000/mm^3$, and no other source or only a "minor" bacterial source on examination had a pneumonia infection as seen on a chest radiograph. A clinical policy by the American College of Emergency Physicians states that a chest radiograph should be considered in children older than 3 months who have a temperature $\geq 39°C$ and a WBC count $\geq 20,000/mm^3$ and that a chest radiograph is usually not indicated in febrile children older than 3 months who have a temperature $\leq 39°C$ without clinical evidence of acute pulmonary disease [90]. The British Thoracic Society similarly recommends that a chest radiograph should be considered in children younger than 5 years old who have a temperature $\geq 39°C$ caused by an unclear source of infection [159]. These recommendations may change based on the decline of the prevalence of pneumococcal pneumonia [160]. No decision rules exist for pediatric pneumonia that help with disposition decisions in children who have pneumonia, but the majority of patients are treated on an outpatient basis. Both amoxicillin (80 mg/kg/d divided twice or three times daily) and macrolide antibiotics (eg, azithromycin, 10 mg/kg by mouth on the first day, then 5 mg/kg/d for 4 more days) are acceptable. Treatment duration is usually from 7 to 10 days (with the exception of azithromycin), but no definitive evidence supports a specific duration of therapy [159].

Future directions and questions

The pneumococcal vaccine has already had a significant impact on the epidemiology of bacterial infection in young children, and this vaccine has already seems to have had some impact on the practice patterns of pediatricians. Pediatricians who were surveyed were found to order fewer blood and urine tests and were less likely to prescribe antibiotics in a hypothetical scenario of an 8-month-old febrile but otherwise healthy infant when the child had been fully immunized with PCV7 compared with a nonimmunized child [161]. Some authors have begun advocating a less aggressive approach to the evaluation of the immunized febrile child, given the decline in invasive pneumococcal disease with PCV7 [131,133]. Other investigators, however, are urging caution before changing evaluation and management strategies, postulating that invasive pneumococcal disease will persist for several reasons: not all serotypes are covered by vaccine, some children will not be able to mount an adequate immune response to form protective antibodies, and some children still will be incompletely immunized [162].

Other questions regarding PCV7 have arisen. Among the seven serotypes, the amount of disease reduction is variable [34–36]. Furthermore, although the overall rate of invasive pneumococcal disease is lower, there is an increase in the percentage of invasive pneumococcal disease caused by nonvaccine serogroups [33–36]. The clinical implications of this serotype replacement remains unclear but will depend on the capacity of the PCV7 vaccine to protect against these noncovered serotypes as well as the virulence of the nonvaccine strains. Pneumococcal conjugate vaccines intended to cover nine and 11 serotypes are in development [163]. Another question that remains unanswered is the duration of protection afforded to patients who are immunized. Finally, the approach to the patient who is not fully immunized is still unclear. Partial immunization likely provides some protection against pneumococcus; the majority of patients in the post-surveillance PCV7 studies were not fully immunized (ie, three vaccinations), but there was still a decline in invasive pneumococcal disease [33].

Despite the use of the PCV7 vaccine, patients will still develop bacteremia, and there will be still be a need for better tests to diagnose invasive bacterial disease. Several additional tests are being studied as potential surrogate markers for bacterial disease in young children: procalcitonin (not yet available in the United States), C-reactive protein, and interleukin-6 [164–171].

Summary

Most children 0 to 36 months of age who have fever without an obvious source have viral infections, but certain subsets of febrile children are at higher risk for more serious bacterial disease. The child who appears to be toxic, regardless of age, needs a comprehensive work-up, antibiotic coverage, and admission to the hospital. Generally, this entails a complete blood count with differential, blood culture, urinalysis and urine culture, lumbar puncture with cerebrospinal fluid analysis, Gram stain and culture, and, when indicated, chest radiographs and stool studies. These patients should receive broad-spectrum parenteral antibiotics before hospital admission. The febrile neonate (0–28 days old) is at high risk for serious bacterial infection, even with benign examination and normal screening laboratory results. Therefore, these patients also need a complete blood count with differential, blood culture, urinalysis and urine culture, lumbar puncture with cerebrospinal fluid analysis, Gram stain and culture, and, when indicated, chest radiographs and stool studies. Febrile neonates should receive empiric antibiotic coverage, typically with ampicillin (50 mg/kg IV, or 100 mg/kg if meningitis is suspected) and cefotaxime (50 mg/kg IV, or 100 mg/kg if meningitis is suspected) or gentamicin (2.5 mg/kg IV).

The febrile young infant (1–3 months old) is also at significant risk for bacterial infection. These patients need complete blood counts, blood cultures, urinalyses and urine cultures. A lumbar puncture with cerebrospinal fluid analysis, Gram stain, and culture should be strongly considered because laboratory tests such as the white blood cell count are inaccurate in predicting which patients have meningitis. When they are clinically indicated, chest radiographs and stool studies should be obtained as well. If any of these test findings are abnormal (including peripheral WBC $\geq$ 15,000/mm^3 or $\leq$ 5000/mm^3, band-to-neutrophil ratio $\geq$ 0.2, a urine dipstick test positive for nitrite or leukocyte esterase, or $\geq$ 5 WBCs/hpf, or organisms seen on Gram stain; cerebrospinal fluid with $\geq$ 8 WBC/mm^3 or organisms on Gram stain; or $\geq$ 5 WBC/hpf on the stool specimen or evidence of pneumonia on a chest radiograph), these patients should receive ceftriaxone (50 mg/kg IV or IM, or 100 mg/kg IV if meningitis is suspected)

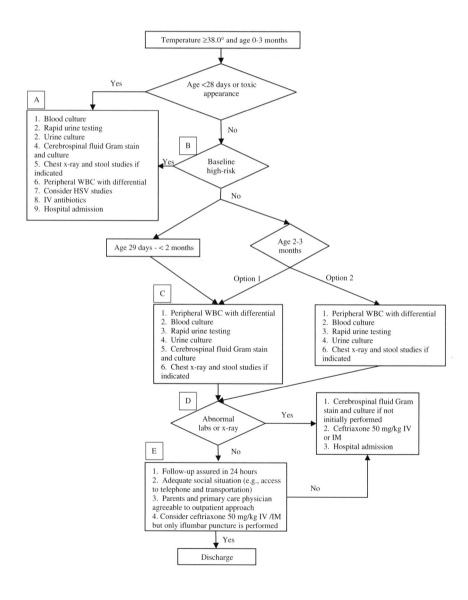

and should be admitted to the hospital. If these initial laboratory results are normal, a patient can be discharged if follow-up within 24 hours (or sooner if clinically worse) can be assured. The administration of ceftriaxone, 50 mg/kg IV or IM, should be considered if a lumbar puncture is performed, but if a lumbar puncture is not performed, antibiotics should be withheld. If a patient is 2 to 3 months old and the practitioner is comfortable with pediatric assessment skills, these children can be treated similarly to older febrile children.

The older infant or toddler (3–36 months old) who has a temperature of $\geq 39.0°C$ may be treated more selectively. In this age group, if no febrile source is identified definitively, a catheterized urine specimen for evaluation (dipstick, urinalysis, microscopy, or Gram stain) and urine culture should be obtained in girls less than 2 years old, if two or more of the following risk factors are present: age less than 12 months old, fever for 2 or more days, temperature $\geq 39.0°C$, white, and no alternative source of fever. All boys younger than 6 months old and all uncircumcised boys younger than 12 months old should also have catheterized urine sent for rapid urine testing and culture. Based on pre-PCV7 data, the most cost-effective approach to the child who has not had at least three PCV7 doses is to obtain a CBC. If the WBC count is $\geq 15,000/mm^3$, a blood culture should be ordered and the administration of ceftriaxone should be considered. Other options (eg, blood culture only or CBC and blood culture with selective antibiotic administration) are reasonable. However, in nontoxic children who have had three PCV7 immunizations and who are not at risk for meningococcal disease, some practitioners believe that obtaining any blood work is unnecessary. The current

Fig. 1. (*A*) Urine testing can be accomplished either by microscopy, Gram stain, or urine dipstick. Chest radiographs are indicated in patients with hypoxia, tachypnea, abnormal lung sounds, or respiratory distress. Stool studies are indicated in patients with diarrhea. Herpes simplex virus testing should be considered in the presence of risk factors (see text for details). HSV testing is best accomplished by polymerase chain reaction or viral culture. Neonates should receive both ampicillin (50 mg/kg IV, or 100 mg/kg IV if meningitis is suspected) and cefotaxime (50 mg/kg, or 100 mg/kg IV if meningitis is suspected) or gentamicin (2.5 mg/kg IV). Additionally, neonates with findings suggestive of HSV infection should receive acyclovir (20 mg/kg IV). Older children should receive ceftriaxone (50 mg/kg IV, or 100 mg/kg IV if meningitis is suspected). A WBC count with differential may be ordered, but the results should not dissuade the clinician from pursuing a full evaluation and treatment with antibiotics. (*B*) Young patients who have increased underlying risk include children who were premature, had prolonged hospital stays after birth, those with underlying medical conditions, patients with indwelling medical devices, fever lasting longer than 5 days, or patients already on antibiotics. (*C*) Urine testing can be accomplished either by microscopy, Gram stain, or urine dipstick. Chest radiographs are indicated in patients with hypoxia, tachypnea, abnormal lung sounds, or respiratory distress. Stool studies are indicated in patients with diarrhea. (*D*) Abnormal laboratory findings: peripheral WBC count $\leq 5,000/mm^3$ or $\geq 15,000/mm^3$ or band-to-neutrophil ratio ≥ 0.2; urine testing, ≥ 5 WBC/hpf, bacteria on Gram stain, or positive leukocyte esterase or nitrite; cerebrospinal fluid, ≥ 8 WBC/mm^3 or bacteria on Gram stain; stool specimen, ≥ 5 WBC/hpf; and chest radiograph, infiltrate detected. (*E*) Administering ceftriaxone (50 mg/kg IV or IM) is optional but should only be considered in patients who have undergone lumbar puncture. Patients who have not undergone lumbar puncture should not get ceftriaxone. (*Adapted from* Baraff L. Management of fever without source in infants and children. Ann Emerg Med 2000;36(6):602–14.)

evidence suggests that this may become a reasonable approach, but studies addressing this specific approach have not yet been published (Figs. 1 and 2).

Finally, it is critically important to recognize that there is no combination of clinical assessment and diagnostic testing that will successfully identify all patients with serious infection at the time of initial presentation. Therefore, the importance of timely reassessment cannot be overemphasized, and caretakers must be instructed to return to the ED or the office immediately for any deterioration in the child's condition. While strategies such as that described above may help guide the evaluation and treament of febrile young infants,

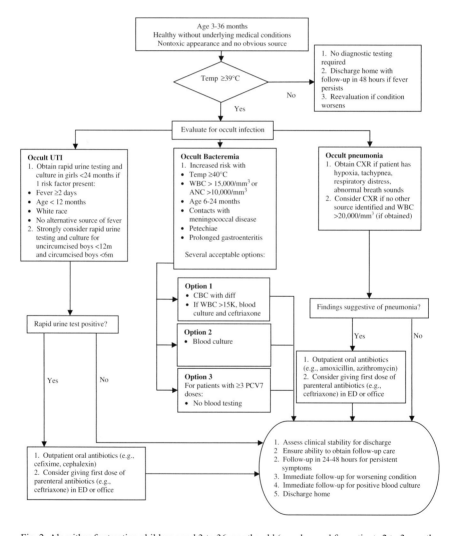

Fig. 2. Algorithm for treating children aged 3 to 36 months old (may be used for patients 2 to 3 months old as well; see text). (*Adapted from* Baraff L. Management of fever without source in infants and children. Ann Emerg Med 2000;36(6):602–14.)

no single approach can capture the nuances of all febrile young patients. Therefore, this approach should serve as an adjunct to, and not a replacement for clinician judgment.

References

[1] Nelson DS, Walsh K, Fleisher GR. Spectrum and frequency of pediatric illness presenting to a general community hospital emergency department. Pediatrics 1992;90(1 Pt 1):5–10.

[2] Krauss BS, Harakal T, Fleisher GR. The spectrum and frequency of illness presenting to a pediatric emergency department. Pediatr Emerg Care 1991;7(2):67–71.

[3] McCaig LF, Burt CW. National Hospital Ambulatory Medical Care Survey: 2002 emergency department summary. Adv Data 2004;340:1–34.

[4] Wittler RR, Cain KK, Bass JW. A survey about management of febrile children without source by primary care physicians. Pediatr Infect Dis J 1998;17(4):271–7 [discussion: 7–9].

[5] Baraff LJ, Schriger DL, Bass JW, et al. Management of the young febrile child: commentary on practice guidelines. Pediatrics 1997;100(1):134–6.

[6] Belfer RA, Gittelman MA, Muniz AE. Management of febrile infants and children by pediatric emergency medicine and emergency medicine: comparison with practice guidelines. Pediatr Emerg Care 2001;17(2):83–7.

[7] Isaacman DJ, Kaminer K, Veligeti H, et al. Comparative practice patterns of emergency medicine physicians and pediatric emergency medicine physicians managing fever in young children. Pediatrics 2001;108(2):354–8.

[8] Kramer MS, Shapiro ED. Management of the young febrile child: a commentary on recent practice guidelines. Pediatrics 1997;100(1):128–34.

[9] Mackowiak PA. Concepts of fever. Arch Intern Med 1998;158(17):1870–81.

[10] Craig JV, Lancaster GA, Taylor S, et al. Infrared ear thermometry compared with rectal thermometry in children: a systematic review. Lancet 2002;360(9333):603–9.

[11] Craig JV, Lancaster GA, Williamson PR, et al. Temperature measured at the axilla compared with rectum in children and young people: systematic review. BMJ 2000;320(7243):1174–8.

[12] Jean-Mary MB, Dicanzio J, Shaw J, et al. Limited accuracy and reliability of infrared axillary and aural thermometers in a pediatric outpatient population. J Pediatr 2002;141(5):671–6.

[13] Gittelman MA, Mahabee-Gittens EM, Gonzalez-del-Rey J. Common medical terms defined by parents: are we speaking the same language? Pediatr Emerg Care 2004;20(11):754–8.

[14] Banco L, Veltri D. Ability of mothers to subjectively assess the presence of fever in their children. Am J Dis Child 1984;138(10):976–8.

[15] Hooker EA, Smith SW, Miles T, King L. Subjective assessment of fever by parents: comparison with measurement by noncontact tympanic thermometer and calibrated rectal glass mercury thermometer. Ann Emerg Med 1996;28(3):313–7.

[16] Graneto JW, Soglin DF. Maternal screening of childhood fever by palpation. Pediatr Emerg Care 1996;12(3):183–4.

[17] Crocetti M, Moghbeli N, Serwint J. Fever phobia revisited: have parental misconceptions about fever changed in 20 years? Pediatrics 2001;107(6):1241–6.

[18] Schmitt BD. Fever phobia: misconceptions of parents about fevers. Am J Dis Child 1980;134(2):176–81.

[19] Grover G, Berkowitz CD, Lewis RJ, et al. The effects of bundling on infant temperature. Pediatrics 1994;94(5):669–73.

[20] Pantell RH, Newman TB, Bernzweig J, et al. Management and outcomes of care of fever in early infancy. JAMA 2004;291(10):1203–12.

[21] McGowan Jr JE, Bratton L, Klein JO, et al. Bacteremia in febrile children seen in a "walk-in" pediatric clinic. N Engl J Med 1973;288(25):1309–12.

[22] Bisgard KM, Kao A, Leake J, et al. *Haemophilus influenzae* invasive disease in the United States, 1994–1995: near disappearance of a vaccine-preventable childhood disease. Emerg Infect Dis 1998;4(2):229–37.

[23] Wenger JD. Epidemiology of *Haemophilus influenzae* type b disease and impact of *Haemophilus influenzae* type b conjugate vaccines in the United States and Canada. Pediatr Infect Dis J 1998;17(9 Suppl):S132–6.

[24] Schuchat A, Robinson K, Wenger JD, et al. Bacterial meningitis in the United States in 1995: Active Surveillance Team. N Engl J Med 1997;337(14):970–6.

[25] Alpern ER, Alessandrini EA, Bell LM, et al. Occult bacteremia from a pediatric emergency department: current prevalence, time to detection, and outcome. Pediatrics 2000;106(3):505–11.

[26] Lee GM, Harper MB. Risk of bacteremia for febrile young children in the post-*Haemophilus influenzae* type b era. Arch Pediatr Adolesc Med 1998;152(7):624–8.

[27] Robinson KA, Baughman W, Rothrock G, et al. Epidemiology of invasive *Streptococcus pneumoniae* infections in the United States, 1995–1998: opportunities for prevention in the conjugate vaccine era. JAMA 2001;285(13):1729–35.

[28] Whitney CG, Farley MM, Hadler J, et al. Increasing prevalence of multidrug-resistant *Streptococcus pneumoniae* in the United States. N Engl J Med 2000;343(26):1917–24.

[29] Kaplan SL, Mason Jr EO, Wald E, et al. Six year multicenter surveillance of invasive pneumococcal infections in children. Pediatr Infect Dis J 2002;21(2):141–7.

[30] American Academy of Pediatrics. Pneumococcal infections. In: Pickering L, editor. Red book: 2003 report of the Committee on Infectious Diseases. 26th edition. Elk Grove Village (IL): American Academy of Pediatrics; 2003. p. 490–500.

[31] Wise RP, Iskander J, Pratt RD, et al. Postlicensure safety surveillance for 7-valent pneumococcal conjugate vaccine. JAMA 2004;292(14):1702–10.

[32] Black S, Shinefield H, Fireman B, et al for the Northern California Kaiser Permanente Vaccine Study Center Group. Efficacy, safety and immunogenicity of heptavalent pneumococcal conjugate vaccine in children. Pediatr Infect Dis J 2000;19(3):187–95.

[33] Black S, Shinefield H, Baxter R, et al for the in Northern California Kaiser Permanente Vaccine Center Group. Postlicensure surveillance for pneumococcal invasive disease after use of heptavalent pneumococcal conjugate vaccine. Pediatr Infect Dis J 2004;23(6):485–9.

[34] Hsu K, Pelton S, Karumuri S, et al. Population-based surveillance for childhood invasive pneumococcal disease in the era of conjugate vaccine. Pediatr Infect Dis J 2005;24(1):17–23.

[35] Whitney CG, Farley MM, Hadler J, et al. Decline in invasive pneumococcal disease after the introduction of protein-polysaccharide conjugate vaccine. N Engl J Med 2003;348(18):1737–46.

[36] Kaplan SL, Mason Jr EO, Wald ER, et al. Decrease of invasive pneumococcal infections in children among 8 children's hospitals in the United States after the introduction of the 7-valent pneumococcal conjugate vaccine. Pediatrics 2004;113(3 Pt 1):443–9.

[37] Alpern E, Henretig F. Fever. In: Fleisher G, Ludwig S, Henretig F, et al, editors. Textbook of pediatric emergency medicine. 5th edition. Philadelphia: Lippincott Williams & Wilkins; 2006. p. 295–306.

[38] Finkelstein JA, Christiansen CL, Platt R. Fever in pediatric primary care: occurrence, management, and outcomes. Pediatrics 2000;105(1 Pt 3):260–6.

[39] Roberts KB. Young, febrile infants: a 30-year odyssey ends where it started. JAMA 2004;291(10):1261–2.

[40] Kuppermann N, Fleisher G, Jaffe D. Predictors of occult pneumococcal bacteremia in young febrile children. Ann Emerg Med 1998;31(6):679–87.

[41] Stanley R, Pagon Z, Bachur R. Hyperpyrexia among infants younger than 3 months. Pediatr Emerg Care 2005;21(5):291–4.

[42] Teach SJ, Fleisher GR for the Occult Bacteremia Study Group. Duration of fever and its relationship to bacteremia in febrile outpatients three to 36 months old. Pediatr Emerg Care 1997;13(5):317–9.

[43] Li SF, Lacher B, Crain EF. Acetaminophen and ibuprofen dosing by parents. Pediatr Emerg Care 2000;16(6):394–7.

[44] McErlean MA, Bartfield JM, Kennedy DA, et al. Home antipyretic use in children brought to the emergency department. Pediatr Emerg Care 2001;17(4):249–51.

[45] Huang SY, Greenes DS. Effect of recent antipyretic use on measured fever in the pediatric emergency department. Arch Pediatr Adolesc Med 2004;158(10):972–6.

[46] Baker MD, Fosarelli PD, Carpenter RO. Childhood fever: correlation of diagnosis with temperature response to acetaminophen. Pediatrics 1987;80(3):315–8.

[47] Baker RC, Tiller T, Bausher JC, et al. Severity of disease correlated with fever reduction in febrile infants. Pediatrics 1989;83(6):1016–9.

[48] Torrey SB, Henretig F, Fleisher G, et al. Temperature response to antipyretic therapy in children: relationship to occult bacteremia. Am J Emerg Med 1985;3(3):190–2.

[49] Yamamoto LT, Wigder HN, Fligner DJ, et al. Relationship of bacteremia to antipyretic therapy in febrile children. Pediatr Emerg Care 1987;3(4):223–7.

[50] Greenes DS, Harper MB. Low risk of bacteremia in febrile children with recognizable viral syndromes. Pediatr Infect Dis J 1999;18(3):258–61.

[51] Smitherman HF, Caviness AC, Macias CG. Retrospective review of serious bacterial infections in infants who are 0 to 36 months of age and have influenza A infection. Pediatrics 2005; 115(3):710–8.

[52] Schutzman SA, Petrycki S, Fleisher GR. Bacteremia with otitis media. Pediatrics 1991;87(1): 48–53.

[53] Turner D, Leibovitz E, Aran A, et al. Acute otitis media in infants younger than two months of age: microbiology, clinical presentation and therapeutic approach. Pediatr Infect Dis J 2002; 21(7):669–74.

[54] DeAngelis C, Joffe A, Willis E, et al. Hospitalization v outpatient treatment of young, febrile infants. Am J Dis Child 1983;137(12):1150–2.

[55] DeAngelis C, Joffe A, Wilson M, et al. Iatrogenic risks and financial costs of hospitalizing febrile infants. Am J Dis Child 1983;137(12):1146–9.

[56] Paxton RD, Byington CL. An examination of the unintended consequences of the rule-out sepsis evaluation: a parental perspective. Clin Pediatr (Phila) 2001;40(2):71–7.

[57] Baker MD, Bell LM. Unpredictability of serious bacterial illness in febrile infants from birth to 1 month of age. Arch Pediatr Adolesc Med 1999;153(5):508–11.

[58] Kadish HA, Loveridge B, Tobey J, et al. Applying outpatient protocols in febrile infants 1–28 days of age: can the threshold be lowered? Clin Pediatr (Phila) 2000;39(2):81–8.

[59] Pena BM, Harper MB, Fleisher GR. Occult bacteremia with group B streptococci in an outpatient setting. Pediatrics 1998;102(1 Pt 1):67–72.

[60] Hoffman JA, Mason EO, Schutze GE, et al. *Streptococcus pneumoniae* infections in the neonate. Pediatrics 2003;112(5):1095–102.

[61] Dagan R, Powell KR, Hall CB, et al. Identification of infants unlikely to have serious bacterial infection although hospitalized for suspected sepsis. J Pediatr 1985;107(6):855–60.

[62] Dagan R, Sofer S, Phillip M, et al. Ambulatory care of febrile infants younger than 2 months of age classified as being at low risk for having serious bacterial infections. J Pediatr 1988;112(3): 355–60.

[63] Jaskiewicz JA, McCarthy CA, Richardson AC, et al for the Febrile Infant Collaborative Study Group. Febrile infants at low risk for serious bacterial infection–an appraisal of the Rochester criteria and implications for management. Pediatrics 1994;94(3):390–6.

[64] Ferrera PC, Bartfield JM, Snyder HS. Neonatal fever: utility of the Rochester criteria in determining low risk for serious bacterial infections. Am J Emerg Med 1997;15(3):299–302.

[65] Baker MD, Bell LM, Avner JR. Outpatient management without antibiotics of fever in selected infants. N Engl J Med 1993;329(20):1437–41.

[66] Baraff L. Management of fever without source in infants and children. Ann Emerg Med 2000;36(6):602–14.

[67] Steere M, Sharieff GQ, Stenklyft PH. Fever in children less than 36 months of age: questions and strategies for management in the emergency department. J Emerg Med 2003;25(2):149–57.

[68] Bonsu BK, Harper MB. Utility of the peripheral blood white blood cell count for identifying sick young infants who need lumbar puncture. Ann Emerg Med 2003;41(2):206–14.

[69] Bonsu BK, Harper MB. Identifying febrile young infants with bacteremia: is the peripheral white blood cell count an accurate screen? Ann Emerg Med 2003;42(2):216–25.

[70] Brown L, Shaw T, Wittlake WA. Does leucocytosis identify bacterial infections in febrile neonates presenting to the emergency department? Emerg Med J 2005;22(4):256–9.

[71] Gorelick MH, Shaw KN. Screening tests for urinary tract infection in children: a meta-analysis. Pediatrics 1999;104(5):e54.

[72] Shaw KN, McGowan KL, Gorelick MH, et al. Screening for urinary tract infection in infants in the emergency department: which test is best? Pediatrics 1998;101(6):E1.

[73] Al-Orifi F, McGillivray D, Tange S, et al. Urine culture from bag specimens in young children: are the risks too high? J Pediatr 2000;137(2):221–6.

[74] Committee on Quality Improvement, Subcommittee on Urinary Tract Infection. Practice parameter: the diagnosis, treatment, and evaluation of the initial urinary tract infection in febrile infants and young children. Pediatrics 1999;103(4):843–52.

[75] Levine DA, Platt SL, Dayan PS, et al. Risk of serious bacterial infection in young febrile infants with respiratory syncytial virus infections. Pediatrics 2004;113(6):1728–34.

[76] Wadsworth SJ, Suh B. In vitro displacement of bilirubin by antibiotics and 2-hydroxybenzoylglycine in newborns. Antimicrob Agents Chemother 1988;32(10):1571–5.

[77] Martin E, Fanconi S, Kalin P, et al. Ceftriaxone–bilirubin-albumin interactions in the neonate: an in vivo study. Eur J Pediatr 1993;152(6):530–4.

[78] Robertson A, Fink S, Karp W. Effect of cephalosporins on bilirubin-albumin binding. J Pediatr 1988;112(2):291–4.

[79] Sadow KB, Derr R, Teach SJ. Bacterial infections in infants 60 days and younger: epidemiology, resistance, and implications for treatment. Arch Pediatr Adolesc Med 1999;153(6):611–4.

[80] Brown JC, Burns JL, Cummings P. Ampicillin use in infant fever: a systematic review. Arch Pediatr Adolesc Med 2002;156(1):27–32.

[81] Brown ZA, Wald A, Morrow RA, et al. Effect of serologic status and cesarean delivery on transmission rates of herpes simplex virus from mother to infant. JAMA 2003;289(2):203–9.

[82] Kimberlin DW, Lin CY, Jacobs RF, et al. Natural history of neonatal herpes simplex virus infections in the acyclovir era. Pediatrics 2001;108(2):223–9.

[83] Kimberlin DW, Lin CY, Jacobs RF, et al. Safety and efficacy of high-dose intravenous acyclovir in the management of neonatal herpes simplex virus infections. Pediatrics 2001;108(2):230–8.

[84] Kimberlin D. Herpes simplex virus, meningitis and encephalitis in neonates. Herpes 2004;11(Suppl 2):A65–76.

[85] Kimberlin DW. Neonatal herpes simplex infection. Clin Microbiol Rev 2004;17(1):1–13.

[86] Chiu CH, Lin TY, Bullard MJ. Identification of febrile neonates unlikely to have bacterial infections. Pediatr Infect Dis J 1997;16(1):59–63.

[87] Baker MD, Avner JR, Bell LM. Failure of infant observation scales in detecting serious illness in febrile, 4- to 8-week-old infants. Pediatrics 1990;85(6):1040–3.

[88] Baskin MN, O'Rourke EJ, Fleisher GR. Outpatient treatment of febrile infants 28 to 89 days of age with intramuscular administration of ceftriaxone. J Pediatr 1992;120(1):22–7.

[89] Baker MD, Bell LM, Avner JR. The efficacy of routine outpatient management without antibiotics of fever in selected infants. Pediatrics 1999;103(3):627–31.

[90] American College of Emergency Physicians Clinical Policies Committee and Subcommittee on Pediatric Fever. Clinical policy for children younger than three years presenting to the emergency department with fever. Ann Emerg Med 2003;42(4):530–45.

[91] Bramson RT, Meyer TL, Silbiger ML, et al. The futility of the chest radiograph in the febrile infant without respiratory symptoms. Pediatrics 1993;92(4):524–6.

[92] Bonsu BK, Harper MB. A low peripheral blood white blood cell count in infants younger than 90 days increases the odds of acute bacterial meningitis relative to bacteremia. Acad Emerg Med 2004;11(12):1297–301.

[93] Shapiro ED, Aaron NH, Wald ER, et al. Risk factors for development of bacterial meningitis among children with occult bacteremia. J Pediatr 1986;109(1):15–9.

[94] Teele DW, Dashefsky B, Rakusan T, et al. Meningitis after lumbar puncture in children with bacteremia. N Engl J Med 1981;305(18):1079–81.

[95] Bonsu BK, Harper MB. Accuracy and test characteristics of ancillary tests of cerebrospinal fluid for predicting acute bacterial meningitis in children with low white blood cell counts in cerebrospinal fluid. Acad Emerg Med 2005;12(4):303–9.

[96] Byington CL, Enriquez FR, Hoff C, et al. Serious bacterial infections in febrile infants 1 to 90 days old with and without viral infections. Pediatrics 2004;113(6):1662–6.

[97] Liebelt EL, Qi K, Harvey K. Diagnostic testing for serious bacterial infections in infants aged 90 days or younger with bronchiolitis. Arch Pediatr Adolesc Med 1999;153(5):525–30.

[98] Titus MO, Wright SW. Prevalence of serious bacterial infections in febrile infants with respiratory syncytial virus infection. Pediatrics 2003;112(2):282–4.

[99] Rittichier KR, Bryan PA, Bassett KE, et al. Diagnosis and outcomes of enterovirus infections in young infants. Pediatr Infect Dis J 2005;24(6):546–50.

[100] Dayan PS, Hanson E, Bennett JE, et al. Clinical course of urinary tract infections in infants younger than 60 days of age. Pediatr Emerg Care 2004;20(2):85–8.

[101] Hoberman A, Wald ER, Hickey RW, et al. Oral versus initial intravenous therapy for urinary tract infections in young febrile children. Pediatrics 1999;104(1 Pt 1):79–86.

[102] Fleisher GR, Rosenberg N, Vinci R, et al. Intramuscular versus oral antibiotic therapy for the prevention of meningitis and other bacterial sequelae in young, febrile children at risk for occult bacteremia. J Pediatr 1994;124(4):504–12.

[103] Teach SJ, Fleisher GR for the Occult Bacteremia Study Group. Efficacy of an observation scale in detecting bacteremia in febrile children three to thirty-six months of age, treated as outpatients. J Pediatr 1995;126(6):877–81.

[104] McCarthy PL, Sharpe MR, Spiesel SZ, et al. Observation scales to identify serious illness in febrile children. Pediatrics 1982;70(5):802–9.

[105] Bass JW, Steele RW, Wittler RR, et al. Antimicrobial treatment of occult bacteremia: a multicenter cooperative study. Pediatr Infect Dis J 1993;12(6):466–73.

[106] Kuppermann N. Occult bacteremia in young febrile children. Pediatr Clin North Am 1999;46(6):1073–109.

[107] Lee GM, Fleisher GR, Harper MB. Management of febrile children in the age of the conjugate pneumococcal vaccine: a cost-effectiveness analysis. Pediatrics 2001;108(4):835–44.

[108] Jaffe DM, Tanz RR, Davis AT, et al. Antibiotic administration to treat possible occult bacteremia in febrile children. N Engl J Med 1987;317(19):1175–80.

[109] Harper MB, Bachur R, Fleisher GR. Effect of antibiotic therapy on the outcome of outpatients with unsuspected bacteremia. Pediatr Infect Dis J 1995;14(9):760–7.

[110] Bulloch B, Craig WR, Klassen TP. The use of antibiotics to prevent serious sequelae in children at risk for occult bacteremia: a meta-analysis. Acad Emerg Med 1997;4(7):679–83.

[111] Rothrock SG, Harper MB, Green SM, et al. Do oral antibiotics prevent meningitis and serious bacterial infections in children with Streptococcus pneumoniae occult bacteremia? a meta-analysis. Pediatrics 1997;99(3):438–44.

[112] Rothrock SG, Green SM, Harper MB, et al. Parenteral vs oral antibiotics in the prevention of serious bacterial infections in children with Streptococcus pneumoniae occult bacteremia: a meta-analysis. Acad Emerg Med 1998;5(6):599–606.

[113] Baraff LJ, Oslund S, Prather M. Effect of antibiotic therapy and etiologic microorganism on the risk of bacterial meningitis in children with occult bacteremia. Pediatrics 1993;92(1):140–3.

[114] Stoll ML, Rubin LG. Incidence of occult bacteremia among highly febrile young children in the era of the pneumococcal conjugate vaccine: a study from a children's hospital emergency department and urgent care center. Arch Pediatr Adolesc Med 2004;158(7):671–5.

[115] Yang YJ, Huang MC, Wang SM, et al. Analysis of risk factors for bacteremia in children with nontyphoidal Salmonella gastroenteritis. Eur J Clin Microbiol Infect Dis 2002;21(4):290–3.

[116] Zaidi E, Bachur R, Harper M. Non-typhi Salmonella bacteremia in children. Pediatr Infect Dis J 1999;18(12):1073–7.

[117] Kuppermann N, Malley R, Inkelis SH, et al. Clinical and hematologic features do not reliably identify children with unsuspected meningococcal disease. Pediatrics 1999;103(2):E20.

[118] Wang VJ, Kuppermann N, Malley R, et al. Meningococcal disease among children who live in a large metropolitan area, 1981–1996. Clin Infect Dis 2001;32(7):1004–9.
[119] Wang VJ, Malley R, Fleisher GR, et al. Antibiotic treatment of children with unsuspected meningococcal disease. Arch Pediatr Adolesc Med 2000;154(6):556–60.
[120] Mandl K, Stack A, Fleisher G. Incidence of bacteremia in infants and children with fever and petechiae. J Pediatr 1997;131(3):398.
[121] Nielsen HE, Andersen EA, Andersen J, et al. Diagnostic assessment of haemorrhagic rash and fever. Arch Dis Child 2001;85(2):160–5.
[122] Wells LC, Smith JC, Weston VC, Collier J, et al. The child with a non-blanching rash: how likely is meningococcal disease? Arch Dis Child 2001;85(3):218–22.
[123] American Academy of Pediatrics. Committee on Infectious Diseases. Prevention and control of meningococcal disease. recommendations for use of meningococcal vaccines in pediatric patients. Pediatrics 2005;116(2):496–505.
[124] Bachur R, Harper MB. Reevaluation of outpatients with *Streptococcus pneumoniae* bacteremia. Pediatrics 2000;105(3 Pt 1):502–9.
[125] Bandyopadhyay S, Bergholte J, Blackwell CD, et al. Risk of serious bacterial infection in children with fever without a source in the post-*Haemophilus influenzae* era when antibiotics are reserved for culture-proven bacteremia. Arch Pediatr Adolesc Med 2002;156(5):512–7.
[126] Norberg A, Christopher NC, Ramundo ML, et al. Contamination rates of blood cultures obtained by dedicated phlebotomy vs intravenous catheter. JAMA 2003;289(6):726–9.
[127] Waltzman ML, Harper M. Financial and clinical impact of false-positive blood culture results. Clin Infect Dis 2001;33(3):296–9.
[128] Thuler LC, Jenicek M, Turgeon JP, et al. Impact of a false positive blood culture result on the management of febrile children. Pediatr Infect Dis J 1997;16(9):846–51.
[129] DeAngelis C, Joffe A, Wilson M, et al. Iatrogenic risks and financial costs of hospitalizing febrile infants. Am J Dis Child 1983;137(12):1146–9.
[130] Evidence based clinical practice guideline for outpatient management of fever of uncertain source in children 2 to 36 months of age. 2003. Available at http://www.cincinnatichildrens.org/svc/alpha/h/health-policy/ev-based/feverii.htm. Accessed August 1, 2005.
[131] Kuppermann N. The evaluation of young febrile children for occult bacteremia: time to reevaluate our approach? Arch Pediatr Adolesc Med 2002;156(9):855–7.
[132] Baraff LJ, Bass JW, Fleisher GR, et al for the Agency for Health Care Policy and Research. Practice guideline for the management of infants and children 0 to 36 months of age with fever without source. Ann Emerg Med 1993;22(7):1198–210.
[133] Baraff LJ. Clinical policy for children younger than three years presenting to the emergency department with fever [editorial]. Ann Emerg Med 2003;42(4):546–9.
[134] Green S, Rothrock S. Evaluation styles for well-appearing febrile children: are you a "risk-minimizer" or a "test-minimizer"? Ann Emerg Med 1999;33(2):211–4.
[135] Hoberman A, Chao HP, Keller DM, et al. Prevalence of urinary tract infection in febrile infants. J Pediatr 1993;123(1):17–23.
[136] Shaw KN, Gorelick M, McGowan KL, et al. Prevalence of urinary tract infection in febrile young children in the emergency department. Pediatrics 1998;102(2):E16.
[137] Bachur R, Harper MB. Reliability of the urinalysis for predicting urinary tract infections in young febrile children. Arch Pediatr Adolesc Med 2001;155(1):60–5.
[138] Gorelick MH, Shaw KN. Clinical decision rule to identify febrile young girls at risk for urinary tract infection. Arch Pediatr Adolesc Med 2000;154(4):386–90.
[139] Gorelick MH, Hoberman A, Kearney D, et al. Validation of a decision rule identifying febrile young girls at high risk for urinary tract infection. Pediatr Emerg Care 2003;19(3):162–4.
[140] Schoen EJ, Colby CJ, Ray GT. Newborn circumcision decreases incidence and costs of urinary tract infections during the first year of life. Pediatrics 2000;105(4 Pt 1):789–93.
[141] Task Force on Circumcision. Circumcision policy statement. Pediatrics 1999;103(3):686–93.
[142] Zorc JJ, Kiddoo DA, Shaw KN. Diagnosis and management of pediatric urinary tract infections. Clin Microbiol Rev 2005;18(2):417–22.

[143] Huicho L, Campos-Sanchez M, Alamo C. Metaanalysis of urine screening tests for determining the risk of urinary tract infection in children. Pediatr Infect Dis J 2002;21(1):1–11.

[144] Wubbel L, Muniz L, Ahmed A, et al. Etiology and treatment of community-acquired pneumonia in ambulatory children. Pediatr Infect Dis J 1999;18(2):98–104.

[145] Margolis P, Gadomski A. Does this infant have pneumonia? JAMA 1998;279(4):308–13.

[146] Jadavji T, Law B, Lebel MH, et al. A practical guide for the diagnosis and treatment of pediatric pneumonia. CMAJ 1997;156(5):703.

[147] Lynch T, Platt R, Gouin S, et al. Can we predict which children with clinically suspected pneumonia will have the presence of focal infiltrates on chest radiographs? Pediatrics 2004; 113(3 Pt 1):E186–9.

[148] Rothrock SG, Green SM, Fanelli JM, et al. Do published guidelines predict pneumonia in children presenting to an urban ED? Pediatr Emerg Care 2001;17(4):240–3.

[149] Leventhal JM. Clinical predictors of pneumonia as a guide to ordering chest roentgenograms. Clin Pediatr (Phila) 1982;21(12):730–4.

[150] Taylor JA, Del Beccaro M, Done S, et al. Establishing clinically relevant standards for tachypnea in febrile children younger than 2 years. Arch Pediatr Adolesc Med 1995;149(3): 283–7.

[151] Zukin DD, Hoffman JR, Cleveland RH, et al. Correlation of pulmonary signs and symptoms with chest radiographs in the pediatric age group. Ann Emerg Med 1986;15(7):792–6.

[152] Mower WR, Sachs C, Nicklin EL, et al. Pulse oximetry as a fifth pediatric vital sign. Pediatrics 1997;99(5):681–6.

[153] Tanen DA, Trocinski DR. The use of pulse oximetry to exclude pneumonia in children. Am J Emerg Med 2002;20(6):521–3.

[154] Davies HD, Wang EE, Manson D, et al. Reliability of the chest radiograph in the diagnosis of lower respiratory infections in young children. Pediatr Infect Dis J 1996;15(7):600–4.

[155] McCarthy PL, Spiesel SZ, Stashwick CA, et al. Radiographic findings and etiologic diagnosis in ambulatory childhood pneumonias. Clin Pediatr (Phila) 1981;20(11):686–91.

[156] Courtoy I, Lande AE, Turner RB. Accuracy of radiographic differentiation of bacterial from nonbacterial pneumonia. Clin Pediatr (Phila) 1989;28(6):261–4.

[157] Swingler GH, Hussey GD, Zwarenstein M. Randomised controlled trial of clinical outcome after chest radiograph in ambulatory acute lower-respiratory infection in children. Lancet 1998; 351(9100):404–8.

[158] Bachur R, Perry H, Harper MB. Occult pneumonias: empiric chest radiographs in febrile children with leukocytosis. Ann Emerg Med 1999;33(2):166–73.

[159] British Thoracic Society of Standards of Care Committee. BTS Guidelines for the management of community acquired pneumonia in childhood. Thorax 2002;57:1–24.

[160] Black SB, Shinefield HR, Ling S, et al. Effectiveness of heptavalent pneumococcal conjugate vaccine in children younger than five years of age for prevention of pneumonia. Pediatr Infect Dis J 2002;21(9):810–5.

[161] Lee KC, Finkelstein JA, Miroshnik IL, et al. Pediatricians' self-reported clinical practices and adherence to national immunization guidelines after the introduction of pneumococcal conjugate vaccine. Arch Pediatr Adolesc Med 2004;158(7):695–701.

[162] Klein JO. Management of the febrile child without a focus of infection in the era of universal pneumococcal immunization. Pediatr Infect Dis J 2002;21(6):584–8 [discussion: 613–4].

[163] O'Brien KL, Santosham M. Potential impact of conjugate pneumococcal vaccines on pediatric pneumococcal diseases. Am J Epidemiol 2004;159(7):634–44.

[164] Fernandez Lopez A, Luaces Cubells C, Garcia Garcia JJ, et al. Procalcitonin in pediatric emergency departments for the early diagnosis of invasive bacterial infections in febrile infants: results of a multicenter study and utility of a rapid qualitative test for this marker. Pediatr Infect Dis J 2003;22(10):895–903.

[165] Galetto-Lacour A, Zamora SA, Gervaix A. Bedside procalcitonin and C-reactive protein tests in children with fever without localizing signs of infection seen in a referral center. Pediatrics 2003;112(5):1054–60.

[166] Gendrel D, Raymond J, Coste J, et al. Comparison of procalcitonin with C-reactive protein,

interleukin 6 and interferon-alpha for differentiation of bacterial vs. viral infections. Pediatr Infect Dis J 1999;18(10):875–81.

[167] Hsiao AL, Baker MD. Fever in the new millennium: a review of recent studies of markers of serious bacterial infection in febrile children. Curr Opin Pediatr 2005;17(1):56–61.

[168] Isaacman DJ, Burke BL. Utility of the serum C-reactive protein for detection of occult bacterial infection in children. Arch Pediatr Adolesc Med 2002;156(9):905–9.

[169] Pulliam PN, Attia MW, Cronan KM. C-reactive protein in febrile children 1 to 36 months of age with clinically undetectable serious bacterial infection. Pediatrics 2001;108(6):1275–9.

[170] van Rossum AM, Wulkan RW, Oudesluys-Murphy AM. Procalcitonin as an early marker of infection in neonates and children. Lancet Infect Dis 2004;4(10):620–30.

[171] Carrol ED, Newland P, Riordan FA, et al. Procalcitonin as a diagnostic marker of meningococcal disease in children presenting with fever and a rash. Arch Dis Child 2002;86(4): 282–5.

ELSEVIER
SAUNDERS

PEDIATRIC CLINICS
OF NORTH AMERICA

Pediatr Clin N Am 53 (2006) 195–214

Pediatric Ear, Nose, and Throat Emergencies

Morgen Bernius, MD[a],*, Donna Perlin, MD[b]

[a]*Department of Surgery, Division of Emergency Medicine,
University of Maryland School of Medicine, 110 Sout Paca Street, Sixth Floor, Suite 200,
Baltimore, MD 21201, USA*
[b]*Division of Pediatric Emergency Medicine, Department of Pediatrics,
University of Maryland Hospital for Children, 22 South Greene Street, Baltimore, MD 21201, USA*

Acute otitis media (AOM) is the most common infection for which antibiotics are prescribed in children, resulting in more than 20 million antibiotic prescriptions annually. New practice guidelines published by the American Academy of Pediatrics and the American Academy of Family Physicians [1] call for the judicious use of antibiotics in view of increasing antibiotic resistance and the unclear necessity of the use of antibiotics in children with uncomplicated AOM. These guidelines are reviewed below. In addition, this article reviews several other common ear, nose, and throat (ENT) entities, including sinusitis and dental emergencies, and current strategies in diagnosing and treating these conditions.

Acute otitis externa

Otitis externa is an inflammation of the external auditory canal and external surface of the tympanic membrane, which can be caused by a variety of conditions that compromise the lining of the canal. The ear canal is lined with squamous epithelial cells and cerumen glands that provide a lipid protective barrier [2]. When the skin of the ear canal is exposed to water for long periods, it becomes macerated and desquamates, causing the development of microfissures. The protective cerumen is washed away and the pH level of the ear canal changes [3]. Otitis externa is, therefore, seen frequently in swimmers, hot and humid climates, and in conditions that lead to water retention in the ear such as pro-

---

* Corresponding author.
E-mail address: morgen2131@aol.com (M. Bernius).

doi:10.1016/j.pcl.2005.10.002
pediatric.theclinics.com

longed showers. In addition, the skin of the canal can be disrupted by local trauma such as foreign bodies, cotton swabs, insect bites, and eczema. Other predisposing factors include hearing aids, earplugs, and an immunocompromised host.

Otitis externa is characterized by otalgia, ranging from an initial pruritus to severe pain, which is worse with motion or chewing. Pain is reproduced by pulling on the auricle or tragus. The canal becomes erythematous and increasingly swollen, leading to a sensation of aural fullness and possible hearing loss. Treatment should include cleansing and debridement of the ear canal with a cotton swab and hydrogen peroxide or Burow's solution. An acidifying agent (2% acetic acid) is useful to inhibit the growth of bacteria and fungi. Topical antibiotic drops alone or mixed with antifungal agents or steroids (to decrease inflammation) should be continued for at least 3 days after the resolution of symptoms. A cotton wick of gauze strip may be required to allow diffusion of the drops into the edematous ear canal. Nonsteroidal anti-inflammatory drugs (NSAIDs) or even opiates may be required for pain control. Cultures are not necessary unless the condition is refractory to treatment [4].

There are multiple types of otitis externa, including furunculosis (localized inflammation), diffuse bacterial otitis externa ("swimmer's ear"), otomycosis (fungal infection), and malignant or necrotizing otitis externa [4]. Each involves inflammation of the ear canal.

Furunculosis is a localized form of otitis externa, in which an abscess develops in a hair follicle with spreading of the infection to the surrounding skin. This usually occurs in the outer third of the ear canal. The most common causative agent is *Staphylococcus aureus*. Treatment includes the incision and drainage of pointing, fluctuant abscesses and the application of topical antistaphylococcal antibiotics.

Diffuse bacterial otitis externa, the most common type, is also known as swimmer's ear because of its most common predisposing factor. With prolonged exposure to water, the ear canal becomes colonized with gram-negative bacteria. *Pseudomonas aeruginosa* is the pathogen that most commonly causes diffuse bacterial otitis externa [4]. The initial symptom is usually pruritus that becomes increasingly painful as the infection progresses. Increasing erythema and edema of the auditory canal lead to a feeling of pressure and may lead to conductive hearing loss. Secretions may be scant serous to profuse and purulent. Systemic symptoms are usually absent.

Otomycosis, a chronic superficial infection of the ear canal, the tympanic membrane, or both is relatively rare and tends to occur in the tropics, in an immunocompromised host, or from prolonged topical steroid or antibiotic usage [2,4]. It may be primary or secondary. In primary fungal infection, the most common causative agent is *Aspergillus* organisms, which cause 80% to 90% of otomycosis infections [4]. It may also be caused by *Candida* organisms. The appearance of the debris in the canal can suggest a fungal infection because it has a peppered appearance secondary to black mycelial elements [4]. The most common presenting complaint with primary otomycosis is intense pruritus. Secondary otomycosis, which is a fungal infection superimposed on an existing bacterial infection, tends to present with intense pain. Treatment consists of applying topical antifungal agents such as clotrimazole or itraconazole [2], which may be combined with a topical steroid or an acidifying agent.

Malignant or necrotizing otitis externa is an advanced case of otitis externa presenting with tender preauricular lymphadenopathy, protrusion of a swollen auricle, and possible cellulitis of the skin over the mastoid bone [3]. There is severe erythema, edema, and tenderness of the ear canal and surrounding structures associated with intense pain and otorrhea. Facial nerve palsy may occasionally accompany malignant otitis externa, with possible involvement of other cranial nerves [4]. It is most commonly caused by *P aeruginosa* and is often a complication of persistent otitis externa. Treatment requires systemic antibiotics, including oral ciprofloxacin, ofloxacin, or intravenous antipseudomonal drugs. Prolonged therapy is usually required [4]. Imaging with CT is often helpful to define the bone involvement and extent of disease, and follow-up CT scans are useful to follow the efficacy of treatment. ENT referral is recommended.

Prevention of otitis externa may be achieved by thoroughly drying the ear canal after bathing and swimming and instilling a 2% acetic acid solution or any of the over-the-counter swimmer's eardrops. The use of earplugs may also reduce infection in swimmers.

Acute otitis media

AOM is a closed-space inflammatory process in the middle ear, associated with a middle ear effusion (MEE), signs and symptoms of middle ear inflammation, and a recent, abrupt onset of clinical symptoms [1]. AOM is the most common infection for which antibiotics are prescribed in children, resulting in more than 20 million antibiotic prescriptions annually [1]. It has a prevalence that peaks at 6 to 20 months of age and has a propensity to become chronic and recurrent [5].

AOM must be differentiated from otitis media with effusion (OME), a nonsuppurative, secretory otitis media. Although OME may predispose to and may succeed AOM, it does not have an infectious component and, therefore, should be considered separately. AOM tends to occur with greater frequency in the first 2 years of life, possibly related to the immaturity of immunologic defenses and eustachian tube function and structure and perhaps to the greater proportions of time spent in the horizontal position [5]. It tends to occur more frequently in males and in Native American or Inuit populations [5]. It has been associated with lower socioeconomic status, possibly because of crowding, poor hygiene, suboptimal nutrition, and to limited access to health care and medical resources. Breastfeeding has been found to have a protective effect [5], whereas exposure to tobacco smoke and repeated exposure to other children, such as at a daycare facility, have been related to an increase in propensity toward the disease. Children who have craniofacial anomalies and Down syndrome have an increased prevalence of AOM [5].

The presence of a viral upper respiratory infection may lead to the development of AOM secondary to associated eustachian tube dysfunction, associated nasopharyngeal bacterial colonization, and damage to the respiratory tract epithelium with subsequent impairment of mucociliary clearance of bacteria [2]. Pathogenic bacteria can be isolated from middle ear aspirates in approximately 70% of cases of AOM [5]. The three most common causative pathogens are *Streptococcus pneumoniae*, nontypable *Haemophilus influenzae*, and *Moraxella catarrhalis* [1,5]. A small number of cases involve group A streptococci, *Staph aureus*, and gram-negative organisms. Although viruses may be isolated from middle ear exudates, it is uncertain whether they can cause AOM without a bacterial co-pathogen [5].

The clinical presentation of AOM may be highly variable, especially in infants and toddlers. AOM may present with a history of an abrupt onset of otalgia, irritability, otorrhea, or fever. The presence of bulging of the tympanic membrane (TM) has the highest positive predictive value for the existence of MEE [1], followed by limited or absent mobility of the TM and air-fluid levels noted on otoscopy [1]. The TM may be erythematous or opacified.

The American Academy of Pediatrics and The American Academy of Family Physicians (AAP/AAFP) Clinical Practice Guideline specifies that the diagnosis of AOM meet all three requirements of rapid onset, the presence of MEE, and the presence of signs and symptoms of middle ear inflammation [1]. These same guidelines call for the judicious use of antibiotics in view of increasing antibiotic resistance and the unclear necessity of the use of antibiotics in children with uncomplicated AOM. Guidelines advocate the option of a period of observation without the use of antimicrobial agents for 48 to 72 hours in selected children with uncomplicated AOM. These cases include children from 6 months to 2 years of age with nonsevere illness if the diagnosis of AOM is uncertain and children older than 2 years of age with nonsevere illness, despite the certainty of the diagnosis of AOM. If the patient fails to improve with symptomatic treatment within 48 to 72 hours, the guidelines recommend that the patient be reassessed and antibiotic therapy initiated [1].

A recent study from the United Kingdom [6] compared a group of children aged 6 months to 10 years who received the observation option with a similar group of children who received immediate antibiotics. The authors found that 76% of children in the observation group never required antimicrobials. The immediate use of antibiotics was associated with a 1-day reduction of illness but no difference in school absence or pain scores.

If the decision is made to treat AOM with antibiotics, amoxicillin is recommended by the AAP/AAFP guidelines at a dosage of 80 to 90 mg/kg/d [1]. Patients who are allergic to penicillin may alternatively be treated with azithromycin, clarithromycin, or erythromycin-sulfisoxazole. A course of 10 days is recommended for children younger than 6 year of age [7]. If the illness is severe or amoxicillin treatment has failed, amoxicillin-clavulanate, 90 mg/kg/d, would be the antimicrobial of choice to increase the coverage for β-lactamase-producing *H influenzae* and *M catarrhalis* [8].

In the patient who is vomiting, a single dose of ceftriaxone, 50 mg/kg, given intramuscularly, has been shown to be effective in the treatment of AOM [9,10]. The patient who has failed amoxicillin-clavulanate therapy may be considered for treatment with a 3-day course of parenteral ceftriaxone [10] or, alternatively, a course of oral clindamycin [1].

Foreign bodies of the nose and ear

Foreign bodies are a relatively common occurrence in the pediatric population. A wide variety of objects have been retrieved from both the ear and nose, including toys, food, paper, beads, and insects. The child may present with a clear history of foreign body self-insertion or, alternatively, may present with recurrent epistaxis, foul odor, or pain in the ear or nose. Impairment in hearing [11] or olfaction may be the presenting complaint. Many children are asymptomatic, and the foreign body is discovered by a parent or a physician during a routine examination.

Physical findings may vary with the duration of the foreign body impaction, the size of the foreign body, and the physical characteristics of the foreign body itself. In the case of a small object that has been inserted very recently, the child may be asymptomatic, whereas with a large foreign body, the child may present with evidence of local trauma. An insect in the ear canal often presents with intense, constant pain and a sensation of movement in the ear. A child with a chronic foreign body may present with unilateral nasal or otic discharge, a foul odor, or recurrent epistaxis secondary to chronic irritation [12].

Special mention should be made of battery impactions. Children can easily insert small batteries from electronic devices (eg, calculators, handheld video games, or watches) into their nostrils. Button batteries may release small amounts of chemicals and voltage that may lead to alkaline chemical burns, necrosis, or septal–tympanic perforation [13]. Batteries should be removed as soon as possible to prevent these complications [12].

The removal of nasal or otic foreign bodies should only be attempted in the emergency department if there is reasonable expectation for removal because repeated, failed attempts result in increased swelling and trauma and possibly repositioning the object into a less favorable location [12]. The child needs to be restrained adequately or sedated, and all necessary supplies should be readily available, including a good light source, nasal speculum, alligator forceps, a curette, suction apparatus, and a topical vasoconstrictor to reduce tissue edema before attempt at removal [12]. Foreign body removal may be accomplished by manually grasping the object with forceps, getting behind the object with a curette or irrigation, or by applying suction to the surface of the foreign body.

The physical characteristics of the foreign body as well as the anatomic location should be considered before removal is attempted [12]. A live insect will be most easily removed if it is first killed with either 2% lidocaine or mineral oil. Irrigation should be avoided with objects such as vegetable matter or sponges because the added water will make the foreign body swell, impeding its extraction [12]. A smooth round foreign body that completely occludes the orifice is not likely to be removed successfully with a curette or forceps and may benefit from suction. Positive pressure ventilation with either a bag-valve mask or mouth-to-mouth pressure from the caregiver while occluding the noninvolved nostril has been successful in the removal of large, occlusive nasal foreign bodies [14]. Foreign bodies that are unable to be removed in the emergency department should be referred to an otolaryngologist for removal. Oral antibiotics are recommended in this situation to prevent infection of the obstructed orifice [12].

Epistaxis

The nose has a rich vascular supply, making it vulnerable to episodes of bleeding, either spontaneously or as a result of localized trauma. Most of the time, the bleeding is mild and self-limited, although it can be profuse and life threatening. In the pediatric population, epistaxis is most commonly the result of local trauma from nose picking or a recent upper respiratory infection [15]. Other causes include facial trauma, foreign bodies, cocaine or heroin sniffing, or sinusitis. Less commonly, systemic causes such as hepatic disease, leukemia, idiopathic thrombocytopenia, or coagulopathies may be associated with epistaxis. Coagulopathies may be congenital, such as von Willebrand's disease, hemophilia, and Osler-Weber-Rendu disease, or acquired (NSAIDs, aspirin, and rat poison) [15].

Epistaxis can be classified according to location of bleeding in the nasal cavity as either anterior or posterior. Anterior bleeding accounts for approximately 90% of episodes of epistaxis [16] and usually arises from a venous vascular plexus on the anterior nasal septum, known as Kiesselbach's plexus. The mucosa overlying Kiesselbach's plexus is fragile and firmly adhered to the cartilage of the septum, making it prone to trauma. Because the bleeding is mostly from capillary or venous sources, anterior bleeds tend to be characterized by a slow, persistent oozing [16]. Posterior bleeds, however, originate from the sphenopalatine artery in the posterior nasal cavity and nasopharynx [17] and tend to bleed more profusely. This type of bleeding carries a higher risk of airway compromise, aspiration of blood, and life-threatening hemorrhage [16].

Epistaxis tends to occur with a bimodal incidence [17]. Episodes that occur in the 2- to 10-year-old category are more frequently minor anterior bleeds, whereas bleeding that occurs in the second peak of those over the age 50 years is more likely to be more severe posterior bleeding [15]. Most cases of epistaxis require minimal intervention. Mild epistaxis without active bleeding requires only recommendations to minimize the recurrence of bleeding, including limiting local trauma (eg, no nose blowing or picking) and applying nasal hydration with saline mist or ointments and increasing ambient humidity with a cool mist vaporizer to reduce mucosal irritation.

If minor bleeding recurs, the patient (or parent) may be instructed to pinch the nostrils together for 5 to 30 minutes nonstop (without frequent peeking to see if

Physical examination is guided by the mechanism of trauma and suspicion for associated injuries. A thorough neurologic examination should always be performed because dental injuries are a subset of head trauma. The most important aspects of the focused dental examination include palpation, percussion, and mobility evaluation. Adjacent soft tissues should be evaluated for injury and embedded tooth fragments.

Radiographic examination

Children with dental fractures, luxation, tooth pain, or discoloration after a traumatic injury should undergo dental radiography. Radiographs can show the degree of tooth displacement and indicate a root or bony fracture or permanent tooth bud displacement [33].

Dental fractures

Infraction
A tooth infraction is defined as an incomplete fracture or crack of the enamel, without a loss of tooth structure. Physical examination and radiographic findings are normal. No intervention is required other than reassurance. Complications are rare [34].

Uncomplicated crown fracture
An uncomplicated crown fracture is defined as a fracture to the enamel (or enamel and dentin) that does not involve the pulp. These are type 1 and 2 fractures in the Ellis classification system (Table 1). On physical examination, the yellow dentin may be visualized. Bleeding, significant pain, or pink, exposed pulp is not present. Urgent dental consultation is unnecessary for such injuries. Management consists of filing down rough edges of small fractures and attempting to restore tooth structure in larger fractures. Successful treatment depends on the degree of dentin exposure and the presence of concomitant injury to the periodontal ligament [34].

Complicated crown fracture
A complicated crown fracture, or Ellis type 3 fracture, involves the enamel, dentin, and pulp. Prompt dental care is required when pulp is exposed to prevent further injury and infection. In primary teeth, decisions on management are based

Table 1
Ellis classification of tooth fractures

Classification	Involvement
Type 1	Enamel only
Type 2	Enamel and dentin
Type 3	Enamel, dentin, and pulp
Type 4	Root involvement

on the life expectancy of the tooth and on the degree of pulpal damage. Pulpal treatment options for permanent teeth include pulp capping and partial or complete pulpectomy [34]. Successful treatment depends on the duration of pulp exposure, the degree of dentin exposure, and the stage of root development.

Root fracture

Root fractures involve the cementum, dentin, and pulp. On clinical examination, the coronal fragment is mobile and attached to the gingiva, which may be displaced. Radiographic evidence of one or more horizontal fracture lines may be seen. Radiographic diagnosis may be difficult in a primary tooth if the succedaneous tooth is overlying. Primary teeth may be left in place if the fracture is in the apical third of the tooth and the crown segment is stable. However, if the fracture is in the middle or coronal third of the tooth, extraction is necessary because of the instability of the crown segment and the potential for infection from saliva contamination of the exposed pulp [35]. Treatment for permanent teeth with root fractures involves urgent repositioning and stabilization of the coronal fragment to allow healing of the periodontal ligament and neurovascular supply. The prognosis for permanent tooth root fractures is not affected by the location of the fracture. Pulp necrosis from displacement of the coronal segment occurs in 25% of patients with root fractures [34].

Luxation injuries

Luxation is displacement of a tooth from its normal position. Luxation injury to a permanent tooth is a true dental emergency, and immediate management is necessary to maintain the viability of an injured periodontal ligament.

Subluxation

Subluxation injury occurs when a tooth is abnormally loosened but not displaced, causing injury to the supporting periodontal ligament. On physical examination, the tooth is mobile and may exhibit sulcal bleeding. Radiographic study findings are normal. No intervention is required for primary teeth, other than dental follow-up. Permanent teeth should be stabilized and splinted as needed for comfort. The prognosis is good, but dental follow-up is necessary because pulpal necrosis may occur in cases in which the neurovascular supply is damaged [34].

Lateral luxation

Lateral luxation injury occurs when a tooth is displaced in a nonaxial direction, causing damage to the periodontal ligament and possible contusion or fracture of the supporting alveolar bone. On physical examination, the tooth is displaced laterally, with the crown usually directed palatally or lingually. The tooth may not be tender and is often immobile and trapped in its new position. Radiographic examination shows an increase in the periodontal ligament space and apical tooth displacement, with possible associated alveolar bone fracture.

Primary teeth may be allowed to reposition passively or may be actively repositioned and splinted, unless the injury is severe or the life expectancy of the tooth is short. Permanent teeth require immediate active repositioning and splinting. Long-term risks include pulp necrosis and progressive root resorption [34].

Intrusion

Intrusion injury occurs when a tooth is driven apically and displaced into the alveolar bone, causing compression injury to the periodontal ligament and often fracturing the bony socket. On physical examination, the tooth appears shortened or, in severe cases, missing. It is immobile and nontender to the touch. Radiographic examination can visualize the apical displacement of the tooth as well as any disruption in the periodontal ligament. The treatment for intruded primary teeth is to allow spontaneous re-eruption, unless the tooth has been displaced into the succeeding permanent tooth. Permanent teeth may be repositioned actively or passively, depending on the degree of intrusion and maturity of the root apex. In permanent teeth with less mature roots, spontaneous re-eruption may be allowed. There is a high risk of pulp necrosis and root resorption in intrusion injuries to permanent teeth with mature root apices [34].

Extrusion

In extrusion injury, the tooth is displaced apically from the socket, resulting in damage to the periodontal ligament and the neurovascular supply. On physical examination, the tooth appears longer than adjacent teeth and is mobile. Radiographic examination shows a widening of the apical periodontal ligament space. Primary teeth may be extracted or repositioned. Permanent teeth should be urgently repositioned and stabilized to allow healing of the periodontal ligament and to maintain the integrity of the neurovascular supply. These patients must also be followed closely because they are at high risk for pulp necrosis [34].

Avulsion injuries

Tooth avulsion is the complete displacement of the tooth from its socket, severing the periodontal ligament. The prognosis for tooth survival is indirectly related to the time spent out of the oral cavity, with 85% to 97% survival at 5 minutes and near zero survival at 1 hour [36]. Avulsed primary teeth should not be replanted. Permanent teeth, however, should be replanted as soon as possible. The patient does not need to wait for professional medical assistance, and with proper guidance, the tooth can be replanted by the first capable person, such as the patient, a parent, or coach. The tooth should be handled by the crown to avoid damaging the periodontal ligament. Debris may be removed by gentle rinsing with saline or water, but scrubbing should be avoided. The tooth may then be replanted and held in place by biting down on a gauze pad (or by gentle finger pressure) until a splint can be placed by a medical or dental professional. If the tooth cannot be replanted within 5 minutes, it may be stored in a culture medium to preserve the vitality of periodontal ligament cells. The American Academy of

Pediatric Dentistry recommends (in order of preference) the use of Viaspan, Hanks' balanced salt solution, cold milk, saliva, physiologic saline, or water. Milk is the preferred substance most readily available. The avulsed tooth may also be placed in a container of the child's saliva. Transport of the tooth in the child's mouth is not recommended because of risks of aspiration or further damage to the tooth. Close dental follow-up is necessary to evaluate for tooth survival. Tetanus prophylaxis and antibiotic coverage should be considered [34].

Cervical lymphadenopathy

Cervical lymphadenopathy is one of the most common clinical problems encountered in any pediatric primary care or emergency practice. Although cervical lymphadenopathy may herald the presence of a more serious systemic disease or malignancy, it is most often a normal and temporary response to a benign and localized infection. The dilemmas for the emergency physician are distinguishing between benign and severe causes of lymphadenopathy and initiating the proper investigation of the more perilous cases.

Lymphadenopathy is defined by the presence of nodal tissue measuring more than 1 cm in diameter [37]. This enlargement may be caused by proliferation of normal lymphocytes and macrophages in response to an antigen (eg, viral infection), infiltration of the lymph node by inflammatory cells in response to an infection of the node (lymphadenitis), proliferation within the lymph node of neoplastic lymphocytes or macrophages (lymphoma), or nodal infiltration with metabolite-loaded histiocytes in the storage diseases (eg, Gaucher and Nieman-Pick diseases).

The anterior cervical chain drains the mouth and pharynx and is the most common site of lymph node enlargement, resulting from common upper respiratory viral and bacterial infections. The posterior cervical chain and occipital nodes are most often enlarged in response to infection or dermatitis of the scalp. Generalized lymphadenopathy is defined as lymph node enlargement in two or more noncontiguous regions, including the liver and spleen. The discovery of enlarged cervical nodes should always prompt a complete examination of the remaining nodal regions to determine if it is a localized or systemic response.

History and physical examination

The differential diagnosis of cervical lymphadenopathy is quite broad (Box 1). The examination of the enlarged lymph nodes for tenderness, warmth, erythema, fluctuance, and mobility can yield clues to their cause. Most often, however, the associated findings on history and physical examination provide the salient information. A history of fever, rhinorrhea, sore throat, and cough or evidence of intraoral infection on physical examination are the most common findings in patients with cervical lymphadenopathy arising from an upper respiratory

---

Box 1. Differential diagnosis of cervical lymphadenopathy

Viral

Rhinovirus, parainfluenza virus, influenzavirus, respiratory syn-
cytial virus (RSV), coronavirus, adenovirus, Epstein-Barr virus
(EBV), cytomegalovirus (CMV), rubella virus, rubeola, HSV,
HIV, coxsackievirus

Bacterial

Staphylococcus and *Streptococcus* spp, anaerobes, *Bartonella
henselae*, *Mycobacterium tuberculosis*

Protozoal

Toxoplasmosis

Malignancies

Leukemia, lymphoma, neuroblastoma, rhabdomyosarcoma

Other

Kawasaki disease, collagen vascular disease

---

or intraoral infection. Historical factors that suggest the possibility of chronic
diseases include malnutrition, weight loss, fever, and night sweats. Malignancy
should be suspected in patients with anorexia, weight loss, or fevers and night
sweats or lymphadenitis that is unresponsive to antibiotic treatment. Enlarged
lymph nodes in patients with malignancies are usually nontender, firm, and
rubbery and may be matted together. The presence of associated hepatospleno-
megaly or bruises and petechiae also indicate potential malignancy.

Differential diagnosis

   The most common cause of cervical lymphadenopathy is reactive intranodal
cellular proliferation in response to an upper respiratory infection. Acute bilateral
lymphadenitis is most often caused by the common upper respiratory tract viral
infections, including rhinovirus, parainfluenza virus, influenza virus, RSV, coronavirus, and adenovirus [38]. Bilateral cervical lymphadenopathy is also found
commonly in streptococcal pharyngitis and infectious mononucleosis. Unilateral suppurative lymphadenitis is more likely to be caused by a bacterial in-

fection with *Staph aureus*, group A β-hemolytic streptococci, or other anaerobic organisms in patients with mucositis, gingival infections, or dental abscesses [38].

Viral infections that cause generalized lymphadenopathy, such as EBV and CMV may present initially with bilateral cervical lymphadenitis. Other causes of generalized lymphadenopathy include HIV, rubella virus, varicella-zoster virus, HSV, measles, and coxsackievirus [37].

Causes of subacute and chronic lymphadenopathy include *B henselae* infection (cat-scratch disease), toxoplasmosis (most commonly presenting in the posterior chain), HIV, atypical mycobacteria, *M tuberculosis*, and the nontuberculous mycobacterial infections.

Malignancy must always be considered when evaluating cervical lymphadenopathy. The cervical lymph nodes are the most common site of presentation of malignant tumors of the head and neck. In children ages 6 and younger, the most common malignant causes of enlarged cervical nodes include neuroblastoma, leukemia, rhabdomyosarcoma, and non-Hodgkin's lymphoma. In children older than 6 years, the most common causes are Hodgkin's lymphoma, non-Hodgkin's lymphoma, leukemia, and rhabdomyosarcoma.

Nonsuppurative cervical lymphadenopathy (with at least one node measuring greater than 1.5 cm) is one of the five diagnostic criteria for Kawasaki disease. The others include bilateral bulbar conjunctival injection without exudates, erythematous mouth and pharynx, strawberry tongue with red, cracked lips, generalized erythematous rash, and changes in the peripheral extremities, consisting of either induration and erythema or desquamation. For the diagnosis, patients should have four of these five features as well as fever for at least 5 days' duration [39].

Management

In patients who have cervical lymphadenopathy and no physical findings or historical factors suggesting malignancy or serious systemic disease, observation with primary care follow-up is a reasonable care plan. Patients who have more worrisome findings warrant a more complete work-up. Initial evaluation should consist of a complete blood count with differential, erythrocyte sedimentation rate or C-reactive protein level, placement of a purified protein derivative tuberculin skin test, and plain chest radiography to evaluate for the presence of a mass, pulmonary disease, or mediastinal lymphadenopathy. Primary care or inpatient evaluation may also include serologic testing for EBV, CMV, and HIV infection. For patients who are suspected of having leukemias, pediatric hematology-oncology should be consulted to arrange bone marrow aspiration. Other testing may be guided by clinical suspicion, such as in cases of suspected mononucleosis or cat-scratch disease.

Patients who have a suspected bacterial lymphadenitis should be treated with oral antibiotics with staphylococcal and streptococcal coverage. Fine needle aspiration of a fluctuant node may be performed to guide antibiotic coverage. Patients who have a dominant lymph node of unknown cause that persists for more than 6 weeks or a lymph node that does not respond to antibiotic therapy require surgical referral for lymph node biopsy to rule out malignancy [40].

References

[1] American Academy of Pediatrics and American Academy of Family Physicians. Clinical practice guideline: diagnosis and management of acute otitis media. Pediatrics 2004;113:1451–65.

[2] Marx JA. Extenal otitis. In: Marx JA, editor. Rosen's emergency medicine: concepts and clinical practice. 5th edition. St. Louis (MO): Mosby; 2002. p. 932–3.

[3] Schwartz RH. Otitis externa. In: Long SS, editor. Principles and practice of pediatric infectious diseases. 2nd edition. Orlando (FL): Churchill Livingstone; 2003. p. 199–200.

[4] Eason JV. Otitis externa (PTG). In: Braunwald E, editor. Ferri's clinical advisor: instant diagnosis and treatment. St. Louis (MO): Mosby; 2005. p. 584–5.

[5] Paradise JL. Otitis media. In: Behrman RE, editor. Nelson textbook of pediatrics. 17th edition. Philadelphia: WB Saunders; 2004. p. 2138–49.

[6] Little P, Gould C, Williamson I, et al. Pragmatic randomized controlled trial of two prescribing strategies for childhood otitis media. BMJ 2001;322:336–42.

[7] Dowell SF, Butler JC, Giebink SG. Acute otitis media: management and surveillance in an era of pneumococcal resistance: a report from the Drug-Resistant *Streptococcus pneumoniae* Therapeutic Working Group. Pediatr Infect Dis J 1999;18:1–9.

[8] Dagan R, Hoberman A, Johnson C. Bacteriologic and clinical efficacy of high dose amoxicillin/clavulanate in children with acute otitis media. Pediatr Infect Dis J 2001;20:829–37.

[9] Green SM, Rothrock SG. Single-dose intramuscular ceftriaxone for acute otitis media in children. Pediatrics 1993;91:23–30.

[10] Leibovitz E, Piglansky I, Raiz S, et al. Bacteriologic and clinical efficacy of one day vs. three day intramuscular ceftriaxone for treatment of nonresponsive acute otitis media in children. Pediatr Infect Dis J 2000;19:1040–5.

[11] Mantooth R, Hooker E. Foreign bodies, ear. Available at: http://www.emedicine.com/emerg/topic185.htm. Accessed January 27, 2006.

[12] Barkin RM. Foreign body in the ear and nose. In: Barkin RM, editor. Pediatric emergency medicine: concepts and clinical practice. 2nd edition. St. Louis (MO): Mosby; 1997. p. 729–32.

[13] Palmer O. Button battery in the nose: an unusual foreign body. J Laryngol Otol 1994;108:871–2.

[14] Finkelstein JA. Oral ambu-bag insufflation to remove unilateral nasal foreign bodies. Am J Emerg Med 1996;14:57–8.

[15] Massick D, Tobin E. Otitis media. In: Cummings CW, editor. Otolaryngology: head and neck surgery. 4th edition. St. Louis (MO): Mosby; 2005. p. 4446–7.

[16] Gluckman W, Barricella R. Epistaxis. Available at: http://www.emedicine.com/ped/topic1618.htm. Accessed January 27, 2006.

[17] Evans J, Rothenhaus T. Epistaxis. Available at: http://master.emedicine.com/emerg/topic806.htm. Accessed January 27, 2006.

[18] Wald ER. Sinusitis. Pediatr Ann 1998;27(12):811–8.

[19] American Academy of Pediatrics. Appropriate use of antimicrobial agents. In: Pickering LK, editor. Red book: 2003 report of the Committee on Infectious Diseases. 26th edition. Elk Grove Village (IL): American Academy of Pediatrics; 2003. p. 696.

[20] Diament MJ. The diagnosis of sinusitis in infants and children: x-ray, computed tomography, and magnetic resonance imaging: diagnostic imaging of pediatric sinusitis. J Allergy Clin Immunol 1992;90(3 Pt 2):442–4.

[21] Wald ER, Chiponis D, Ledesma-Medina J. Comparative effectiveness of amoxicillin and amoxicillin-clavulanate potassium in acute paranasal sinus infections in children: a double-blind, placebo-controlled trial. Pediatrics 1986;77:795–800.

[22] Whitley RJ, Roizman B. Herpes simplex viral infection. Lancet 2001;357:1513–8.

[23] Patel NJ, Sciubba J. Oral lesions in young children. Pediatr Clin North Am 2003;50(2):469–86.

[24] Rodu B, Mattingly G. Oral mucosal ulcers: diagnosis and management. J Am Dent Assoc 1992;123:83–6.

[25] American Academy of Pediatrics. Herpes simplex. In: Pickering LK, editor. Red book: 2003 report of the Committee on Infectious Diseases. 26th edition. Elk Grove Village (IL): American Academy of Pediatrics; 2003. p. 344–53.

[26] Amir J, Harel L, Smetana Z, et al. Treatment of herpes simplex gingivostomatitis with acyclovir in children: a randomized double-blind placebo controlled study. BMJ 1997;314:1800–3.

[27] Whitley RJ, Gnann JW. Acyclovir: a decade later. N Engl J Med 1992;327:782–9.

[28] Flores MT. Traumatic injuries in the primary dentition. Dent Traumatol 2002;18:287–98.

[29] Wilson S, Smith GA, Preisch J, et al. Epidemiology of dental trauma treated in an urban pediatric emergency department. Pediatr Emerg Care 1997;13:12.

[30] Kaste LM, Gift HC, Bhat M, et al. Prevalence of incisor trauma in persons 6–50 years of age: United States, 1988–1991. J Dent Res 1996;75:696–705.

[31] Jessee SA. Orofacial manifestations of child abuse and neglect. Am Fam Physician 1995; 52:1829.

[32] Lane WG. Diagnosis and management of physical abuse in children. Clin Fam Pract 2003; 5(2):493–514.

[33] Nelson LP, Shusterman S. Emergency management of oral trauma in children. Curr Opin Pediatr 1997;9:242.

[34] American Academy of Pediatric Dentistry. American Academy of Pediatric Dentistry clinical guideline on management of acute dental trauma. Pediatr Dent 2004;26(7):120–7.

[35] Wilson CF. Management of trauma to primary and developing teeth. Dent Clin North Am 1995;39:133.

[36] Andreasen JO, Borum MK, Jacobsen HL, et al. Replantation of 400 avulsed permanent incisors: diagnosis of healing complications. Endod Dent Traumatol 1995;11:51–8.

[37] Leung AK, Robson WL. Childhood cervical lymphadenopathy. J Pediatr Health Care 2004;18(1):3–7.

[38] Peters TR, Edwards KM. Cervical lymphadenopathy and adenitis. Pediatr Rev 2000;21: 399–405.

[39] American Academy of Pediatrics. Kawasaki syndrome. In: Pickering LK, editor. Red book: 2003 report of the Committee on Infectious Diseases. 26th edition. Elk Grove Village (IL): American Academy of Pediatrics; 2003. p. 392–5.

[40] Brown RL, Azizkhan RG. Pediatric head and neck lesions. Pediatr Clin North Am 1998;45: 889–905.

ELSEVIER
SAUNDERS

PEDIATRIC CLINICS
OF NORTH AMERICA

Pediatr Clin N Am 53 (2006) 215–242

Airway Infectious Disease Emergencies

Keyvan Rafei, MD*, Richard Lichenstein, MD

*Pediatric Emergency Department, University of Maryland Hospital for Children,
22 South Greene Street, Baltimore, MD 21201, USA*

Upper and lower respiratory infections are commonly encountered in the emergency department (ED). Visits for respiratory disease account for 10% of pediatric emergency department visits and 20% of all pediatric hospital admissions [1]. The causes of upper airway infections include croup, epiglottitis, and retropharyngeal abscess-cellulitis (pharyngitis and peritonsillar abscess are described separately). Lower airway infections arise from bacterial and viral infections and cause illnesses such as pneumonia and bronchiolitis. Signs and symptoms overlap with upper and lower airway infections but differentiation is important for the appropriate treatment of these conditions. This article reviews the various clinical characteristics of upper and lower airway infections.

Upper airway infections

Upper airway infections in children include a variety of common and uncommon conditions that can pose significant diagnostic and therapeutic challenges. These difficulties tend to be augmented by the potential for rapid airway compromise and limited evaluations in smaller, apprehensive children. As with many infections, the primary challenge in these conditions lies in identifying the causative pathogen and determining the extent of disease progression. In this discussion, upper airway infections are grouped into the three categories of pharyngotonsillar, laryngotracheobronchial, and deep neck space infections, with an emphasis on recent advances in diagnostic and management strategies.

---

* Corresponding author.
E-mail address: krafei@peds.umaryland.edu (K. Rafei).

0031-3955/06/$ – see front matter © 2006 Elsevier Inc. All rights reserved.
doi:10.1016/j.pcl.2005.10.001   *pediatric.theclinics.com*

Pharyngotonsillar infections

Pharyngotonsillar infections are a group of commonly encountered upper airway problems that include pharyngitis, tonsillitis, and peritonsillar infections. Pharyngitis refers to infections of the pharynx and may also include tonsillitis, in which case the complex is referred to as pharyngotonsillitis. The varied causes but overlapping clinical presentations of these infections have made them the focus of several recent practice guidelines that promote selective and targeted antibacterial therapy in an attempt to reduce the number of unnecessary antibiotic prescriptions [2,3].

Viruses are the most common cause of pharyngitis and tonsillitis in all age groups. Common viral pathogens include respiratory viruses such as influenza virus, parainfluenza virus, adenovirus, and rhinoviruses as well as others, such as coxsackievirus, echoviruses, and Epstein-Barr virus. Group A streptococci (GAS) is the most common bacterial cause of pharyngitis, but a number of other bacteria such as *Mycoplasma pneumoniae*, *Chlamydia pneumoniae*, *Neisseria gonorrhea*, and *Arcanobacterium haemolyticum* are also implicated, although less commonly [2,4,5].

GAS pharyngitis is the only commonly occurring form of bacterial pharyngitis that definitely requires antibiotic therapy [2]. The significance of GAS infection is related to its association with both suppurative complications such as otitis media, sinusitis, peritonsillar and retropharyngeal abscesses and non-suppurative sequelae, including acute rheumatic fever and acute glomerulonephritis [6]. In light of this, the primary challenge in the diagnosis of pharyngitis lies in distinguishing between streptococcal and nonstreptococcal infections.

Clinical symptoms suggestive of GAS infection include the acute onset of sore throat, fever, headache, pain on swallowing, abdominal pain, nausea, vomiting, scarletiniform rash, and enlarged tender anterior cervical lymph nodes [6,7]. Symptoms more suggestive of nonstreptococcal pharyngitis include concurrent viral respiratory or gastrointestinal infection and associated cough, coryza, conjunctivitis, and diarrhea [6]. A number of decision rules have been proposed to assist with the clinical diagnosis of GAS pharyngitis [8–10]. Of these rules, the Centor criteria, which include tonsillar exudates, swollen and tender anterior cervical lymph nodes, lack of cough, and a history of fever, are used most commonly [9]. However, despite their value in stratifying the risk of GAS infection, the sensitivity and specificity of these criteria are too low to forgo the use of diagnostic tests [2,6,11].

Diagnostic tests for the detection of GAS pharyngitis include rapid antigen detection testing (RADT) and blood agar plate cultures of throat swab specimens with adequate pharyngeal and tonsillar secretions. Several authors have shown that the sensitivity of RADT is not fixed but variable and is proportionately related to the pretest clinical likelihood of GAS pharyngitis [12,13]. The higher sensitivity of RADT in adults with a high pretest clinical likelihood of GAS pharyngitis has been used as a justification to forgo culture confirmation in those with negative RADT results [2]. However, unlike adults, the sensitivity of RADT in children, even in those with a higher clinical likelihood of GAS pharyngitis, has been shown to be too low to forgo culture confirmation of negative RADT results [2,12,14].

The use of RADT in patients who are clinically suspected of having GAS pharyngitis has the advantage of rapid availability of results which allows for early treatment, reduction in risk of spread, sooner return to school or work, and reduction in acute morbidity [15]. Additionally, negative RADT with pending culture confirmation allows physicians to withhold antibiotics from the majority of patients who may have an infection from a viral cause [16]. Interestingly, the use of two throat swabs versus one did not increase the sensitivity of a specific RADT, in one study [17]. Laboratory studies such as serum C-reactive protein, peripheral white blood cell (WBC) counts, and erythrocyte sedimentation rates have not been shown to help in differentiating between viral streptococcal sources of infection in acute suppurative tonsillitis [8,18].

In patients who have GAS pharyngitis, antibiotic treatment is indicated for eradicating GAS from the throat, shortening clinical course, decreasing the risk of transmission, and reducing the risk of suppurative sequelae. Furthermore, if started within 9 days after the onset of acute illness, antibiotic therapy has been shown to prevent acute rheumatic fever [6]. Despite the wide variety of antibiotics that have been shown to be effective against GAS, penicillin continues to be the drug of choice. The advantages of oral penicillin V include its proven efficacy, safety, narrow spectrum, and low cost [2,19]. Although the clinical resistance of GAS to penicillins has never been documented, the treatment failure with these agents does occur and are likely related to inadequate compliance with the 3 times daily dosing and 10-day course of therapy [6]. In light of this limitation, some authors have advocated a 10-day single daily dosing regimen of amoxicillin as an equally effective but more convenient alternative for the treatment of GAS pharyngitis [20,21].

Other antibiotic regimens for the treatment of GAS pharyngitis include a single dose of intramuscular penicillin G benzathine as well as various orally administered macrolide and cephalosporin antibiotics. The administration of intramuscular penicillin G avoids the problem of poor compliance but is painful [6]. Erythromycin is recommended for patients who have penicillin allergy, and clindamycin has been shown to be most effective in the elimination of chronic streptococcal carriage [6]. Other antibiotics, most notably azithromycin, have been studied and advocated as 3- and 5-day short-course alternatives to standard penicillin therapy [16,22–24]. The emerging problem of increasing macrolide resistance among GAS bacteria, however, makes this alternative inadvisable [25,26].

The pain associated with pharyngitis can be reduced by the use of standard nonsteroidal anti-inflammatory drugs and acetaminophen [27]. Additionally, children with moderate to severe pharyngitis have been shown to have an earlier onset of pain relief and a shorter duration of sore throat when given a single dose of oral dexamethasone suspension at a dose of 0.6 mg/kg, with a maximum of 10 mg [28].

Laryngotracheobronchial infections

Laryngotracheobronchial infections include a spectrum of common seasonal upper respiratory infections that result from varying degrees of subglottal airway inflammation and obstruction. Laryngotracheobronchitis or croup is most commonly encountered in the second year of life but is also seen frequently in children from the age of 6 months to 6 years. The overall incidence of croup is estimated at 1.5% to 6% and is noted in boys 1.4 to 2 times more commonly than in girls. Admission rates for croup have ranged from 1.5% to 31% and vary greatly with differing practice patterns [29–31].

Parainfluenza virus types 1 and 3 are associated most commonly with croup across all age groups. Other important but less common pathogens include respiratory syncytial virus (RSV), which is noted more commonly in children less than 5 years of age, influenza virus, and *M pneumoniae*, which is more prominent in children older than 5 to 6 years of age. Corresponding to the seasonal prevalence of these pathogens, croup is most predominant in late fall and early winter [6,29].

Characteristic clinical findings of croup include a hoarse voice, inspiratory stridor, and a barking cough, which tends to be worse at night [31]. The severity of these symptoms is related to the degree of narrowing of the larynx and trachea as a result of infection-induced mucosal inflammation and edema [32]. Children with mild croup tend to have inflammation limited to the larynx and present frequently with symptoms of hoarseness, intermittent barky cough, and inspiratory stridor that may be noticeable only with agitation. More severe cases of croup are associated with the extension of inflammation to the trachea and bronchi and present with inspiratory stridor that is audible at rest and is associated with signs of respiratory distress, including nasal flaring and intercostal retractions [32]. Although, croup is diagnosed primarily on clinical grounds, the finding of the classical "steeple sign" in the subglottal area on anteroposterior neck radiographs may be used to confirm the diagnosis [32].

Because of the self-limited nature of croup, the treatment is directed primarily at relieving symptoms of airway obstruction. Standard treatment approaches include the use of humidified air, nebulized racemic epinephrine, and systemic corticosteroids [32]. Although traditional treatment has included a mist of humidified air, a recent randomized controlled study did not show this approach to deliver any incremental benefit in relieving the clinical symptoms in children with moderate croup [32]. The use of nebulized racemic epinephrine, on the other hand, has been well established as an effective, albeit temporary, means of relieving upper airway obstruction by means of local vasoconstriction and decreasing mucosal edema [32–35].

Although the use of racemic epinephrine generally has been reserved for patients who have more severe respiratory distress, the use of systemic oral or intramuscular corticosteroids in the form of dexamethasone has been adopted more commonly and has resulted in a significant reduction in croup-related hospitalizations. Numerous studies have shown that the use of corticosteroids results in a significant reduction of croup-related respiratory symptoms within 6 hours of administration [30,36]. Furthermore, patients treated with corticosteroids have been shown to require fewer doses of racemic epinephrine and have a significant reduction in the duration of emergency department and inpatient stay [30,36]. The addition of inhaled corticosteroids in the form of budesonide to systemic dexamethasone has not been shown to add any incremental benefit to treating children with croup [37]. Other studies have shown that children who have responded to emergency department treatment with nebulized racemic epinephrine and corticosteroids can be safely discharged home after a 2- to 3-hour period of observation [38,39].

Epiglottitis

Epiglottitis, also known as supraglottitis, is an inflammatory condition of the epiglottis and its adjacent structures that can progress rapidly to life-threatening airway obstruction. Compared with adult epiglottitis, the now rare childhood form of this condition presents with several distinctive clinical features that further add to the diagnostic and management challenges of this potentially fatal condition [40,41].

Historically, epiglottitis has been closely associated with invasive *Haemophilus influenzae* type b (Hib) infection. Before the initiation of childhood vaccination programs with Hib-conjugated vaccines in 1998, epiglottitis was second only to meningitis as the most common presentation of Hib disease. Since the early 1990s, a dramatic decline in the number of cases of childhood epiglottitis has been noted [42–47]. By contrast and for uncertain reasons, during this same period, the incidence of epiglottitis in adults has risen significantly [48–50].

In the post-vaccine era, most cases of childhood epiglottitis are caused by pathogens other than *H influenzae*. Among these, *Streptococci* and *Staphylococci* organisms and *Candida albicans* are the most common bacteria, although the relative frequency of epiglottis caused by these pathogens has not increased [43,45,46]. Despite the widespread use of Hib vaccination, a number of cases of Hib-related epiglottitis still have been reported in both immunized and non-immunized children [46,51,52]. For these reasons, an up to date immunization history should not exclude the possibility of epiglottitis in a child with a clinically consistent presentation.

In light of the now infrequent nature of childhood epiglottitis and the potential for rapid clinical deterioration, the diagnosis of this condition requires a high index of suspicion and careful attention to subtle clues in the patient's history and physical examination. Classically, childhood epiglottitis presents as a rapidly progressing illness in a previously healthy individual. Presenting symptoms may include fever, irritability, sore throat, drooling, stridor, and a "hot potato" voice. Additionally, patients frequently appear toxic and exhibit evidence of difficult breathing [46,48,53]. The classic "tripod position" refers to the preferential forward-leaning posture with bracing arms and extension of the neck that allows for maximal air entry. The clinical presentation of childhood epiglottitis differs from that of adults in that the latter tends to have a more gradual course, is less likely to present with airway compromise, and frequently has symptoms that are limited to sore throat and odynophagia [40,41].

Clinical features associated with a higher likelihood of airway obstruction in children include evident respiratory distress, stridor, drooling, and a shorter duration of symptoms [49]. Whenever a child's clinical presentation suggests epiglottitis, priority should be given to protecting the airway. In light of the child's smaller airway, particular care must be taken to avoid advancing a partial airway obstruction to a complete one. For this reason, the clinician should avoid attempts at direct visualization or interventions, such as venopuncture, that may further agitate the patient.

The definitive diagnosis of epiglottitis requires direct visualization of a red swollen epiglottis under laryngoscopy [48,51,53]. Because of the higher likelihood of airway obstruction in children, this examination should be attempted only in an interdisciplinary collaboration with an anesthesiologist and an otolaryngologist in a controlled setting, such as the operating room, which allows for the establishment of an artificial airway.

Once a secure airway has been assured, additional diagnostic and therapeutic interventions can be initiated. Diagnostic studies that can aid in the management of patients who have epiglottitis include a complete blood count (CBC), blood culture, and soft tissue lateral neck radiographs. Patients with epiglottitis have elevated leukocyte counts on complete blood counts and frequently have positive blood cultures for the offending bacterial pathogen [48,51]. Soft tissue lateral neck radiographs may reveal an enlarged epiglottis with a classic "thumbprint" appearance that can confirm the diagnosis in uncertain cases [48].

Broad-spectrum intravenous antibiotics against β-lactamase-producing pathogens should be initiated as soon as a secure airway has been established. The antibiotics most commonly used include ceftriaxone and ampicillin-sulbactam [48]. Although intravenous steroids are frequently administered for the management of airway inflammation, no controlled studies exist to justify this approach in childhood epiglottitis [48].

Differential diagnostic considerations in childhood epiglottitis are extensive and further add to the diagnostic challenges of this condition. Among these, foreign body aspiration or ingestion as well as anaphylactic reactions and laryngotracheobronchial or retropharyngeal infections are most notable. Complications of childhood epiglottitis can include the progression of infection to deep neck tissue as well as respiratory failure and death [48,49,53].

Deep neck space infections

Peritonsillar, retropharyngeal, and parapharyngeal infections are among a group of potentially life-threatening deep neck infections in children that share common clinical features and can present significant diagnostic challenges.

Prompt diagnosis and management of these conditions are essential to ensure successful recovery and prevention of complications [54]. Approaches to the diagnosis and management of these infections are evolving and are the focus of this discussion.

Parapharyngeal and retropharyngeal infections

Parapharyngeal or lateral pharyngeal infections develop in a funnel-shaped space lateral to the pharynx that posteriorly contains the carotid sheath and cranial nerves [55]. In children, these infections may be related to complications of pharyngotonsillar, dental, or adjacent deep neck space infections [55]. Retropharyngeal infections develop in the potential space located between the posterior pharyngeal wall and the prevertebral fascia and may be medical (45%), traumatic (27%), or idiopathic in origin [54,56,57]. Infections secondary to traumatic injuries can be seen in children and adults and may be associated with accidental trauma, foreign body ingestion, or complication of medical procedures [58].

Retropharyngeal infections of medical causes are noted most commonly in children younger than 6 years old, with a peak incidence at 3 years of age [56,58,59]. These infections are generally secondary to contiguous spreading along a lymphatic chain that originates from the nasopharynx, adenoids, and paranasal sinuses and extends to the adjacent pharyngeal tissues. Accordingly, retropharyngeal infections in children tend to be preceded by upper respiratory tract infection such as pharyngitis, tonsillitis, sinusitis, and cervical lymphadenitis. The reduced incidence of retropharyngeal infections in older children has been attributed to the atrophy of these lymphatic structures with age [54,56].

Offending pathogens in these infections tend to vary with the source of origin and frequently include multiple aerobic and anaerobic organisms. Common isolates include *S viridans* and *pyogenes*, *Staph aureus* and *epidermidis*, as well as *Bacteroides*, *Peptostreptococcus*, *Fusobacterium*, *Haemophilus*, and *Klebsiella* organisms [54,56,60]. The extent of tissue involvement can range from cellulitis to frank abscess formation and frequently contributes to the varying clinical presentation.

Because of the relatively infrequent nature of these infections, a high index of clinical suspicion is required to ensure a correct diagnosis and early intervention. The most important clinical findings include fever, neck swelling, pain, and torticollis. A limitation of neck movement associated with decreased oral intake or drooling is an especially important clue in the diagnosis of retropharyngeal abscesses. Other important associated findings include cervical lymphadenopathy and trismus. Interestingly, the signs and symptoms of respiratory distress such as stridor or wheezing are not common initial findings. Important differential diagnostic considerations include epiglottitis, laryngotracheobronchitis, and meningitis [56,58–60].

Once clinical findings raise the possibility of deep neck infections, prompt hematologic and radiologic studies can establish the presence, extent, and location of the infection. Leukocytosis on complete blood count is a common finding and can provide an initial evidence of infection [56,59]. The definitive diagnosis, however, is established with radiologic studies, which most commonly include lateral soft tissue neck radiographs, neck CT, and neck ultrasonography.

Lateral soft tissue neck radiographs can serve as a simple screening study for retropharyngeal infections. Prevertebral soft tissue swelling of greater than 7 mm at the level of the second cervical vertebra or greater than 14 mm at the level of the sixth cervical vertebra is concerning for retropharyngeal pathology. However, unless gas is noted in the area of tissue swelling, distinguishing between cellulitis and abscess formation with this modality is not possible. Additionally, because prevertebral space dimensions can change independently with crying, swallowing, expiration, and neck flexion, best diagnostic results depend on attention to proper technique, which includes imaging during inspiration and with adequate extension [56,59,61]. This requirement can significantly limit the value of neck radiographs in an apprehensive child with limited neck movement.

Because of the limitations associated with radiographs, CT scanning of the neck continues to be the method most commonly used in the diagnosis of deep neck infections. However, although CT scans can be very helpful in assessing the location and extent of infection, the distinction between cellulitis and abscess also may not always be possible. Various studies have reported sensitivities of 43% to 100% and specificities of 57% to 88% for the detection of retropharyngeal abscesses by CT scanning [56,57,59,62]. False-positive reports have been noted with necrotic lymph nodes. In one series, 25% of patients whose condition elicited initial suspicion for abscess formation were at the time of surgical drainage found not to have a pus collection [56,57]. To address this shortcoming, some authors have advocated considering areas of hypodensity greater than 2 cm^3 as more suggestive of abscess formation [63]. Additionally, "scalloping" or the irregularity of the abscess wall on CT scans has been suggested as a late indicator of impending rupture and the need for surgical intervention [64].

Ultrasonography of the neck has been advocated by some authors as a sensitive nonradiating alternative to CT for evaluating deep neck infections as well as monitoring their progression. This modality, especially when combined with color Doppler, can diagnose infections in the early nonsuppurative stage and thereby allow for earlier antibacterial treatment and a reduced number of unnecessary surgeries [56,65,66]. Ultrasonography also has the added benefit of being able to distinguish between adenitis and abscess as well as serve as a tool for guided intraoperative aspiration and drainage [67].

Although the traditional management of deep neck infections had relied more heavily on surgical intervention, more recent evidence suggests that the majority of patients can be managed successfully with early the administration of intravenous antibiotics alone [54,56,58,62,68]. Success rates with a trial of conservative medical management have been reported to be as high as 75% to 90% [56,62]. The selection of the initial antibiotic regimen should be directed by regional bacterial sensitivity patterns and the need for the coverage of multiple mixed aerobic and anaerobic pathogens [56]. Surgical incision and drainage should be reserved for cases that do not respond to medical therapy or those in whom persistent or large abscesses have been noted [54,56,68]. In addition to early antibiotic therapy, careful monitoring and supportive therapy in an institution prepared for airway support can help to ensure successful recovery [54,58, 59,68].

Although rare, complications of deep neck infections in children can pose a serious risk of morbidity and mortality. The complications most commonly reported include airway compromise, aspiration pneumonia, extension of infection to adjacent structures or compartments, and the recurrence of abscesses. Accordingly, most cases of complications are related to inadequately treated abscesses that may result in spontaneous rupture [54,56,58].

Peritonsillar infections

Peritonsillar infection, noted most commonly in patients who have chronic or recurrent tonsillitis, represents an extension of infections from the tonsils [32]. Unlike pharyngitis and tonsillitis, which are noted frequently in all age groups, peritonsillar infections are more common in adolescents and adults [54]. The cause of these infections tends to be polymicrobial and frequently includes both aerobic and anaerobic bacteria [32,54]. Management of these infections is based on their classification into the more common peritonsillar cellulites (PTC) and the less frequent peritonsillar abscesses (PTA) or quinsy [32,69,70].

Typical signs and symptoms of peritonsillar infections include fever, trismus, poor oral intake, drooling, and uvular deviation [32,54,71]. Among these, uvular deviation combined with trismus can aid in differentiating between PTA and PTC [70]. However, because the clinical presentations of PTC and PTA are very similar, the imaging studies are frequently needed to further delineate the degree and extension of infection. CT with contrast enhancement has been the traditional choice for confirmation of abscess formation in children [32,71]. However, some authors have advocated ultrasonography of the neck as a highly sensitive, inexpensive, and nonradiating alternative modality for differentiation between PTC and PTA [72].

The treatment of peritonsillar infections includes antibiotic therapy with or without incision and drainage. Because of their polymicrobial nature and the frequent implication of β-lactamase-producing bacteria, antibiotics with activity against this group of organisms should be selected [54]. Although early antibiotic therapy can abort the formation of an abscess in patients who have peritonsillar cellulites, once pus has formed, an incision and drainage procedure is mandatory [32,54,69,71]. Several studies have found that the incision and drainage of PTAs under conscious sedation in a pediatric emergency department with skilled personnel can be safe and effective [73–75]. Complications of peritonsillar infections include airway obstruction, mediastinitis, and Lemierre syndrome [54,76,77]. The latter is a potentially fatal condition that is usually caused by *F necrophorum* and is characterized by thrombophlebitis of head and neck veins and systemic dissemination of septic emboli [76,78].

Lower airway infections

Definition

Pneumonia has been defined as pulmonary infiltrates as observed on a chest radiograph or by clinical signs and symptoms [79,80]. The World Health Organization considers a diagnosis of pneumonia using clinical signs such as tachypnea (respiratory rate ≥ 50 breaths/min in infants less than 1 year of age and ≥ 40 breaths/min in children more than 1 year of age), retractions, or cyanosis [81,82]. Tachypnea may also be seen in conditions such as asthma and bronchiolitis [83]. Bronchiolitis is defined as an acute lower respiratory tract infection usually in children less than 2 years of age that results in inflammation and obstruction of the peripheral airways [84].

Pathophysiology

Bacterial pneumonia is seen after the inhalation or aspiration of pathogens. Less commonly, it can also occur after hematogenous spread. An inflammatory reaction follows, with the release of fluid and polymorphonuclear white blood cells into the alveoli, followed by fibrin and macrophage deposition over days. Viral pneumonia occurs mainly after the inhalation into the lung of infected droplets from upper airway epithelium. RSV, the major cause of bronchiolitis, is transmitted by contact with infected nasal secretions and more unusually by aerosol spread [84]. In both viral pneumonia and bronchiolitis, the resulting inflammatory response causes epithelial cells to slough into airways, thereby causing bronchial obstruction and hyperinflation. Inflammation mostly affects the smaller caliber peripheral airways, essentially sparing the alveoli in bronchiolitis. Lymphocytes infiltrate in the peribronchial and peribronchiolar epithelium, promoting submucosal and adventitial edema in bronchiolitis. Mucous plugs and cellular debris accumulate because of impaired mucociliary clearance, leading to ball-valve obstruction and subsequent hyperinflation [85]. Viral pneumonia may also predispose infected children to bacterial pneumonia because of damage to mucosal barriers.

Pneumonia in the neonatal period may occur as a result of infection or colonization of the nasopharynx or conjunctiva by organisms found in the mother's vaginal tract. Lung injury from aspiration or host immunologic factors such as in cystic fibrosis [86] may also predispose the child to pneumonia.

Epidemiology

Pneumonia is diagnosed in approximately 4% of children in the United States per year, but the attack rate varies by age. The annual rate of pneumonia is 35 to 40 cases per 1000 children younger than 1 year of age, 30 to 35 cases per 1000 children 2 to 4 years of age, 15 cases per 1000 children aged 5 to 9 years, and less than 10 per 1000 for children older than 9 years of age [79,80,87,88].

Compared with developing nations, most cases of pneumonia in the United States have lower mortality rates and are treated on an outpatient basis [89]. Some populations are at a higher risk for pneumonia, including children who have cystic fibrosis, aspiration syndromes, immunodeficiencies, neurologic impairments, or congenital or acquired pulmonary malformations [90–93]. Bronchiolitis affects nearly all children by the age of 2 years and is the leading cause of hospitalization for infants less than 1 year old. Between 1992 and 2000, bronchiolitis accounted for approximately 1,868,000 ED visits for children less than 2 years of age. For this population in the United States, the overall rate was 26 per 1000 children (95% CI, 22%-31%); the rate of ED visits was 31 per 1000 (95% CI, 26%-36%); and the overall admission rate was 19% [94].

Causes

Many microbiologic agents cause childhood pneumonia, but given the difficulty of establishing the definitive cause, the most likely pathogens are usually inferred from factors such as age, season, and clinical characteristics. Radiographs, blood tests, and cultures are of limited value to the emergency department physician in determining the cause of pneumonia. Depending on the specific laboratory testing used, such as culture, antigen detection, or serology, the microbial cause of pneumonia was found only in 20% to 60% of cases in a European review [95].

S pneumoniae has been found to be the most common cause of bacterial pneumonia and RSV the most common viral cause. In children hospitalized with pneumonia, viral infections become less common with increasing age, whereas the age-specific incidence of bacterial infections remains relatively constant [96]. In both hospitalized and ambulatory children, *S pneumoniae* is the most common bacterial pathogen identified in children less than 4 years of age [97]. RSV infection is most often the cause of bronchiolitis, but contributing pathogens include *Mycoplasma* organisms and other viruses, including parainfluenza virus, influenza virus, rhinovirus, adenovirus, and paramyxovirus (measles) [84].

M pneumoniae and *C pneumoniae* have been isolated more frequently in children 5 to 9 years of age and 10 to 16 years of age, overall [98,99]. Estimates of the percentage of pneumonias caused by *M pneumoniae* vary from 7% to 30% for children 5 to 9 years old to 14% to 51% in children 10 to 16 years old. *C pneumoniae* is implicated less frequently, ranging from 9% to 13% for children 5 to 9 years old to 14% to 35% for children 10 to 16 years old [98,99]. Studies in other areas of the United States have confirmed that *M pneumoniae* and *C pneumoniae* are more common causes of pneumonia in children over 5 years old [100,101].

Overall, *S pneumoniae* causes most cases of bacterial pneumonia in infants and children, and viruses become less prevalent with age, whereas infection from *Mycoplasma* and *Chlamydia* organisms are more commonly found with increasing age, particularly in adolescents. Mixed viral and bacterial infection has been reported in 16% to 34% of children with pneumonia [95,96]. Depending on the clinical picture, the emergency physician should also consider the rarer causes of bacterial pneumonia such as *Staph aureus*, *Moraxella catarrhalis*, *H influenzae* (type b, encapsulated types other than b, and nontypable), group A and B streptococci, *Mycobacterium tuberculosis*, and *Bortadella pertussis* [102].

Clinical characteristics

Streptococcus pneumoniae

The clinical spectrum of signs and symptoms can be broad with pneumonia secondary to *S pneumoniae* infection, ranging from mild, nonspecific symptoms of emesis, cough, and abdominal pain to severe respiratory distress. Tan and colleagues [103] have found the most common presenting symptoms to be fever and nonproductive cough, followed by tachypnea, malaise, lethargy, and rhinorrhea. The most common findings were decreased breath sounds, crackles, or rales. Although the classic finding of radiographic lobar consolidation is often seen, its absence does not eliminate the possibility of pneumococcal pneumonia. In this study, more than half the patients had lobar consolidation, and 38% of patients had effusions. Empyema, a known complication of pneumonia caused by *S pneumoniae*, was present in 14% of the patients.

Antibiotic resistance to *S pneumoniae*, particularly penicillin and cephalosporin resistance, has been noted because the early 1990s. It is an important factor when considering invasive disease and antibiotic selection. As with crude rates of colonization and rates of invasive infection, exposure to antibiotics, young age, and day-care attendance are associated with a greater likelihood of colonization or infection with a penicillin-resistant *S pneumoniae* isolate [104,105]. Serious complications and treatment failures are rare with pneumonia compared with other invasive infections and otitis media [106]. The outcomes of therapy for pneumonia were not found to be different between patients who had penicillin-susceptible and penicillin-nonsusceptible isolates, who were treated with traditional antibiotics [103].

The American Academy of Pediatrics recommends standard antibiotic therapy for noncritically ill, immunocompetent patients who have possible invasive pneumococcal infections other than meningitis. Additional initial broader antibiotic coverage for potential penicillin-nonsusceptible strains could be considered for patients who have lower airway disease who are critically ill, including those with severe multilobar pneumonia with hypoxia. The coverage for possible penicillin- and cefotaxime- or ceftriaxone-nonsusceptible strains could be considered with vancomycin. If vancomycin is used, it should be stopped as soon as antibiotic susceptibilities demonstrate effective alternative agents [106]. Generally, oral therapy with low- or high-dose amoxicillin or second-generation cephalosporins such as cefuroxime should be effective for the initial management of outpatient pneumococcal pneumonia [107] in children less than 5 years of age, excluding the neonatal period. Macrolide antibiotics, including azithromycin, are also appropriate but usually are not necessary given their broad-spectrum coverage [83]. Hospitalized children who are suspected of having pneumococcal pneumonia can be treated with intravenous penicillin, ampicillin, or cefuroxime, unless they are critically ill. Cefotaxime, ceftriaxone, and clindamycin can also be considered when a penicillin-resistant organism is suspected. When a pneumococcal isolate is resistant to cefotaxime or ceftriaxone, clindamycin or vancomycin is recommended [108].

Bronchiolitis

Bronchiolitis is a common, usually self-limited, lower respiratory tract infection caused by RSV that is observed in all geographic areas and usually seen between the months of October through April. There are two strains of RSV, A and B, with numerous genotypes and serotypes. The incubation period varies from 2 to 8 days and, after a prodrome of several days, there is an acute illness characterized by rhinorrhea, cough, and low-grade fever. Young children may be restless or lethargic and drink less than normal. The physical examination is marked by tachypnea, accessory muscle use, wheezes, or crackles. Hypoxemia may be seen secondary to ventilation-perfusion mismatch. The complications of apnea and respiratory failure are seen most frequently in young infants and those with underlying conditions such as prematurity, bronchopulmonary dysplasia, chronic lung disease, congenital heart disease, or immunodeficiencies [84]. In typical cases, laboratory testing or chest radiographs are generally not useful [109] but should be considered if the diagnosis is unclear because viral myocarditis, congenital heart disease, and pneumonia may have similar clinical presentations. Because the diagnosis of bronchiolitis is a clinical one, routine RSV antigen testing has little value in management. Respiratory viral antigen testing may be helpful for infection control if patients are admitted to inpatient units [110]. Oxygen saturation should be performed routinely because cyanosis is difficult to detect and an oxygen saturation of less than 95% was found to be the single best predictor of severe illness in a study of outpatients who had bronchiolitis [111]. The treatment for bronchiolitis is supportive, including intravenous hydration, supplemental oxygen, nasal suction, and mechanical ventilation for respiratory failure [112]. Although many therapies have been attempted for bronchiolitis, including ribavirin, interferon alfa, vitamin A, montelukast, β agonists, epinephrine, and corticosteroids, the optimal therapy is still controversial [113–118]. Although some studies, including a meta-analysis and a systematic review, all failed to show significant clinical improvement with β agonists [116,119], other studies have reported a positive effect [120,121]. Racemic epinephrine may be more effective in the treatment of bronchiolitis because of its additional vasoconstrictor effects in reducing microvascular leakage and mucosal edema. Infants with bronchiolitis, who are treated with nebulized racemic epinephrine, showed more improvement than those treated with nebulized albuterol without an increase in side effects [122,123]. Nebulized ipratropium bromide has not been shown to be of added benefit in treating bronchiolitis [124]. Confounding results have also been seen with corticoste-roids. Although the majority of studies have not demonstrated a benefit with oral, nebulized, or parenteral steroid therapy [125–127], some studies suggest that steroid therapy may be effective in improving recovery [128,129]. In actual hospital practice, short-acting β agonists have been shown to be used 53% to 73% in various studies [94,130]. Steroids are used 8% to 13% [94,130–132]. Many physicians will attempt a trial of nebulized albuterol for children with bron-chiolitis with mild respiratory distress; if there is moderate or severe distress, then nebulized racemic epinephrine and possibly steroids are used. The main-stay of treatment remains supportive care with oxygen and intravenous fluids as needed.

Atypical pneumonia

The term "atypical pneumonia" has referred, for the most part, to pneumonia caused by organisms other than the historically common and more easily cultured bacteria, including most often *M pneumonia, C pneumoniae*, *Chlamydia* species (eg, *burnetti*, *trachomatis*, and *psittaci*), *Legionella pneumophila*, *Bordetella pertussis*, and viral pathogens [102,133,134]. *M pneumoniae and C pneumoniae* have been reported to be the most frequent causes of community-acquired pneumonia in children age 5 years or older [98,99,135].

Pneumonia caused by *C pneumoniae and M pneumoniae* has been reported as relatively mild and rarely resulting in hospitalization; however, *Legionella* spp, which are the exception and are often classified as the causative organisms in atypical pneumonia, usually cause more acute and severe symptoms [134]. The pneumonias caused by *M pneumoniae* and *C pneumoniae* can be further dif-ferentiated clinically by wheezing on presentation [136]. Chest radiographic findings are less likely to be lobar for atypical pneumonias than those caused by *S pneumoniae*. Radiographic abnormalities in *M pneumoniae* vary, but bilateral, diffuse infiltrates are common [137]. Pleural effusions are also less likely to be seen with *M pneumoniae* and *C pneumoniae* [136]. The treatment for atypical pneumonia, covering *M pneumoniae* and *C pneumoniae*, includes macrolide agents in any age group and tetracyclines in children older than 8 years of age. Fluoquinolones (including levofloxacin and oflaxacin but not ciprofloxacin) also are appropriate in children older than 16 years of age [138,139].

Chlamydia trachomatis

C trachomatis can be transmitted from the genital tract of infected mothers to their newborn infants. Following vaginal delivery, 50% of infants will acquire the organism. The nasopharynx and the conjunctivae are the most commonly infected sites, but not all colonized newborns progress to overt infection. Pneu-monia occurs in 5% to 20% of infected infants. *Chlamydia* pneumonia typically presents between 2 and 19 weeks after birth, making *C trachomatis* the most common cause of infection in the 4- to 11-week-old group. A staccato cough, tachypnea, and crackles are often present, but fever is not usually present. Infants who have pneumonia caused by *C trachomatis* often present with bilateral diffuse infiltrates on radiography and peripheral blood eosinophilia. Treatment is initiated based on clinical suspicion; a culture of the nasopharynx or by the detection of bacterial antigens or DNA is confirmatory. A 14-day course of oral erythromycin is recommended but is known to have an efficacy of only 80%. Oral sulfonamides are appropriate in children 2 months old or older [140].

Pertussis

Infection by *B pertussis*, an important respiratory pathogen, may lead to pneumonia. *B pertussis* remains endemic in the United States and continues to cause epidemics, despite widespread vaccination of the population in childhood. However, most cases occur in individuals who have not been adequately vaccinated [141], and infection in vaccinated individuals is usually mild [142]. However the incidence of pertussis among adolescents is rising, and this group forms a reservoir of infection for young infants [143]. A case is defined clinically as an acute cough illness lasting at least 14 days and accompanied by paroxysms of coughing, inspiratory whoop, or post-tussive emesis. If there is exposure to a confirmed case, 14 days of cough is the only requirement for diagnosis [144]. Paroxysmal cough and post-tussive vomiting are the most common presenting symptoms, but fever is rare. In one study, the median age on presentation was 4.1 years; and the overall complication rate was 5.8%, with pneumonia being the most common complication [141]. The complication rate was higher (23.8%) in infants less than 6 months of age. Of all infants less than 6 months of age, the most common complication was apnea (15.9%) [141]. The Red Book reports a fatality rate of 1.3% in children younger than 1 month and 0.3% in children 2 to 11 months of age. Other complications described in a German study include pneumonia (29%) and vomiting (50%) [141]. New seizures occurred in 2% of cases of children less than 1 year of age with pertussis reported to the US Centers for Disease Control and Prevention between 1990 and 1996 [145]. The classic presentation described for pertussis after an incubation period of 7 to 10 days consists of a catarrhal, paroxysmal, and convalescent phase. Young and recently vaccinated children may present atypically. In the catarrhal phase, coryza is present with mild cough lasting 1 to 2 weeks. Fever is absent or low grade, but cough worsens and becomes paroxysmal. These series of coughs may be associated with gagging and cyanosis and last for 2 to 3 weeks before becoming less severe. In the convalescent phase, the cough decreases over weeks to months. Infants with pertussis present atypically, with a short or absent catarrhal phase. Cough with a characteristic whoop is uncommon compared with older children [146]. Children who have been vaccinated and have developed pertussis had cough for a shorter period and less apnea and cyanosis [147]. The clinician should be alerted to the possibility of pertussis based on the typical staccato cough in which multiple forceful coughs proceed in rapid progression followed by a deep inspiration (and possible whooping sound and post-tussive emesis).

These paroxysms may be followed by periods of calm, when the child appears relatively well. Support for the diagnosis of pertussis is a CBC with a high proportion and absolute number ($\geq$ 10,000 lymphocytes/μL) [148]. Young infants should be treated promptly and possibly admitted (given the risk of apnea), based on clinical suspicion, while confirmatory nasopharyngeal cultures are ordered (this will guide prophylaxis of household contacts). Treatment is supportive and includes hydration, nutrition, oxygen, and cardiorespiratory monitoring for complications. Antibiotic treatment during the early often-unrecognized catarrhal stage is required to ameliorate disease, but treatment initiated after paroxysms have been established is still recommended to limit disease spread. The treatment of choice is erythromycin estolate therapy for 14 days, whereas the macrolide agents clarithromycin for 7 days and azithromycin for 5 to 7 days are likely to be effective and better tolerated [149]. Trimethoprim-sulfamethoxazole/SMX is also considered an alternative in children older than 2 months of age [142]. The hospital infection control team and the local public health authorities should be notified of all cases of suspected and confirmed pertussis, and recommendations for the care of exposed people should be followed carefully.

Neonatal pneumonia

Neonatal pneumonia and neonatal sepsis are very different entities than community-acquired pneumonia in older children. These neonates typically present with tachypnea, grunting, and retractions. Nonspecific symptoms such as irritability and poor feeding may also be seen. They may have a fever, or they may present with hypothermia. The most common bacterial agent is group B streptococci, but *Listeria monocytogenes* and other bacteria that cause pneumonia in older infants can also be seen. Gram-negative enteric bacteria can also cause pneumonia in neonates older than 1 week, usually from nosocomial infection [102]. The treatment is supportive and includes broad-spectrum antibiotic coverage such as parenteral ampicillin and gentamicin or ampicillin and cefotaxime.

Diagnosis

Clinical presentation

Pneumonia can have different clinical presentations, depending on the cause and the patient's age. In most cases of bacterial community-acquired pneumonia, children have a sudden onset of fever, tachypnea, and cough. This constellation may be preceded by symptoms of a minor upper respiratory tract infection.

Because neonates may be discharged from the newborn nursery within 24 hours of delivery, the emergency physician may need to identify the neonate who has neonatal pneumonia or neonatal sepsis. These neonates typically present with tachypnea (respiratory rate greater than 60 breaths/min), grunting, and retractions. Nonspecific symptoms such as irritability and poor feeding may also be seen. Hypothermia rather than fever may be seen in this population.

Infants greater than 1 month of age with pneumonia may have similar symptoms, but cough is a more prominent symptom. Unlike newborns, infants who are infected with bacterial pneumonia are more often febrile. Infants with pneumonia caused by viruses or atypical organisms may be afebrile and have wheezing respirations.

Toddlers and preschool children who have pneumonia will usually present with cough, and vomiting, chest pain, and abdominal pain may also be seen. Sometimes, fever and tachypnea may be seen with few other respiratory symptoms [150]. Older children and adolescents may present with symptoms similar to younger children and, in addition, may have generalized symptoms such as headache and abdominal pain. In a study of a series of patients who had bacteremic pneumococcal pneumonia, 28% of patients had no respiratory symptoms, 6% of patients presented with only gastrointestinal symptoms in addition to fever, and 4% of patients had only fever. Tachypnea was recorded in 19% and crackles in 14% of patients [150]. Older children and adolescents may also complain of chest pain, which is often pleuritic in nature and localized [151,152].

In 1997, a Canadian task force [153] reviewed the literature and published evidence-based guidelines for diagnosing pediatric pneumonia. They concluded that the absence of each of four signs (ie, respiratory distress, tachypnea, crackles, and decreased breath sounds) accurately excludes pneumonia (level-2 evidence). When an attempt was made to validate these guidelines in pediatric patients in an urban emergency department, the guidelines were only 45% sensitive (95% CI, 35%-58%) [81] and 66% specific (95% CI, 18%-34%) for diagnosing pneumonia. Positive and negative predictive values were 25% (95% CI, 18%-34%) and 82% (95% CI, 77%-87%), respectively [154]. A recent study has found that patients were more likely to have focal infiltrates on chest radiography if there was a history of fever, tachypnea, increased heart rate, retractions, grunting, crackles, or decreased breath sounds [155]. However this finding still needs to be validated, and a reliable diagnosis of pneumonia is still difficult and requires careful attention to the patient's individual clinical characteristics.

Radiologic and laboratory testing

Chest radiography remains the diagnostic test of choice in tertiary care hospitals, and although they cannot be used to discriminate reliably between bacterial and viral pneumonia [154,156,157], typical patterns are seen. Most radiologists support findings of an alveolar or lobar infiltrate with air bronchograms to be an insensitive but fairly specific indication of bacterial pneumonia [158,159]. Unilobar or round infiltrates may be seen with pneumococcal pneumonia [150,160]. Pneumatoceles may be present with severe necrotizing pneumonia, such as that caused by *Staph aureus* [160]. Viral pneumonia infections usually are characterized by diffuse interstitial infiltrates, hyperinflation, or atelectasis. Peribronchial thickening or hilar adenopathy may also be seen [160,161]. Chest radiographs are often normal in pertussis, but perihilar infiltrates of the right middle lobe or lingual region can also be seen [160]. *Chlamydia* pneumonia is characterized by diffuse interstitial markings and hyperinflation [160,162]. Radiographic findings in patients who are infected with *M pneumoniae* may be normal or have characteristics of viral or bacterial pneumonia as described above. Pleural effusions can also be seen with *M pneumoniae* [160,163] but are more common with *S pneumoniae* and *Staph aureus*. Pediatric tuberculosis can also produce radiographic appearances that vary, which is caused in part by the time point at which the radiograph is taken during the disease's progression. The most common finding is mediastinal or hilar adenopathy. Lobar consolidation as well as pleural effusions can also be seen. In later stages, the classic findings of calcification, focal fibrosis, and cavitary lesions in the upper lobes may be seen, even in children. Miliary tuberculosis is characterized by a diffuse mottling on chest radiographs [164]. Infiltrates may be seen in the right upper lobes for infants and in the posterior or bases of the lung for older children in aspiration syndromes [160].

Other laboratory tests are marginally helpful in distinguishing bacterial from nonbacterial pneumonia. Clinical and epidemiologic factors are most important in reaching a diagnosis; whereas radiographs and selected blood tests can clarify the diagnosis in certain instances [165]. The C-reactive protein level may be elevated in bacterial pneumonia [166,167], and likewise, elevated absolute neutrophil count and elevated white blood cell count are seen frequently with bacterial pneumonia, especially pneumococcal pneumonia [150,168].

Blood cultures are rarely positive in pneumonia because $\leq 10\%$ of children who have pneumonia will have bacteremia, but blood culture results may be helpful in the management of children who are suspected of having pneumococcal pneumonia who do not respond to initial treatment [96,169]. Serologic blood tests are of limited clinical value to the emergency physician. One exception is the cold agglutinin test, which can be performed at the bedside for children over the age of 3 with suspected pneumonia caused by *Mycoplasma*. Although there are false-positive results with viral disease, the test is positive in 70% to 90% of cases of *Mycoplasma* infection [170]. Sputum cultures should be obtained for suspected bacterial pneumonia in preadolescent and adolescent children, but adequate specimens are difficult to obtain in younger children. Many tests performed on nasopharyngeal samples, such as enzyme-linked immunosorbent assays or direct fluorescent antibody assays, are sensitive and specific for detecting viral causes of lower respiratory disease such as respiratory syncytial virus and influenza. Finally, a purified protein derivative skin test should be ordered and a follow-up for reading arranged, if tuberculosis is suspected.

Pulse oximetry measurements of oxygen saturation can correlate with clinical signs of pneumonia (tachypnea and crepitations) in undeveloped countries [171,172] and in areas of high altitude [173]. In developed countries, measurements of oxygen saturation should be useful to the emergency physician in supporting the diagnosis of pneumonia, and influence management decisions such as admission or outpatient treatment.

Treatment

In the ED, the decision to treat a patient for pneumonia is based usually on epidemiologic, clinical, and radiographic findings and other laboratory data as adjuncts. It is unusual for the exact cause to be known at the time of initial treatment. Empiric antibiotic treatment should be based on the likelihood of bacterial disease. For instance, if a virus is detected, usually by rapid antigen detection techniques from a nasopharyngeal aspirate, during a seasonal peak for that virus in a mildly ill child, then withholding antibiotic therapy would be appropriate, despite the presence of a streaky infiltrate on a chest radiograph. However, it is important to recognize that there may be infection with bacterial and viral co-pathogens. Table 1 summarizes the most appropriate first- and second-line therapies for hospitalized and ambulatory pediatric patients who have presumed community-acquired and neonatal pneumonia.

The treatment for lower respiratory illness is supportive and should include supplemental oxygen titrated to an oxygen saturation greater than 95% and albuterol administration by nebulization if wheezing is heard. Intubation and positive pressure ventilation is required for respiratory failure and apnea, which is seen with RSV pneumonia or pertussis. Intravenous fluids should be given to patients who have tachypnea and signs of increased work of breathing or moderate to severe dehydration.

Although many cases of pneumonia can be treated on an ambulatory basis, admission should be considered for patients who have pneumonia who are not responding to outpatient therapy. Empyema may be the cause of prolonged or secondary fever, despite appropriate therapy in a child with pneumonia, and is an important complication of *Staph aureus*, *S pneumoniae*, *H influenzae*, group A *Streptococcus*, *Legionella* organisms, *Mycob tuberculosis*, and other pathogens [174]. All infants younger than 1 month of age should be admitted, and infants under the age of 6 months or children whose caretakers may be poorly compliant with therapy should also be seriously considered for admission. Patients should be admitted to the hospital if there are significant clinical signs such as respiratory distress, dehydration, or hypoxia, but an observation unit in the emergency department can be used if clinical improvement is expected to occur rapidly [175]. Children with other chronic diseases such as congenital heart disease, chronic lung disease, immunodeficiency, or neurologic impairment who present with a new onset respiratory disease are also strong candidates for admission. Finally, patients who have other complications (eg, pneumatoceles) or potential complications (paroxysmal phase of pertussis with apnea) should be admitted for further therapy and observation.

Table 1
Treatment of pediatric pneumonia according to age and causes

Causes and treatment	Age				
	0 – 4 wk	4 – 8 wk	8 – 12 wk	12 wk – 4 y	5 y – adolescence
Causes (in order of prevalence)	Group B streptococci Gram-negative enteric bacterial *L monocytogenes*	*C trachomatis* Viruses (RSV, parainfluenza) *S pneumoniae* *B pertussis* Group B streptococci Gram-negative enteric bacteria *L monocytogenes*	*C trachomatis* Viruses (RSV, parainfluenza) *S pneumoniae* *B pertussis*	Viruses (RSV, parainfluenza, influenza, adenovirus, rhinovirus) *S pneumoniae* *H influenza* (non-b type) *M catarrhalis* Group A streptococci *M pneumoniae* *Mycob tuberculosis*	*M pneumoniae* *C pneumoniae* *S pneumoniae* Viruses (RSV, parainfluenza, influenzavirus, adenovirus, rhinovirus) *Mycob tuberculosis*
Outpatient (in order of initial choice)	—	For *B pertussis* or *Chlamydia* erythromycin or other macrolides	For *B pertussis* or *Chlamydia*, erythromycin or other macrolides, sulfonomides For *S pneumoniae* see next column	Amoxicillin or amoxicillin/clavulante or cefuroxime Macrolides	Macrolides or tetracyclines (≥ 8 y old) Fluoquinolones (≥ 16 y old)
Inpatient	Neonatal pneumonia or sepsis, ceftriaxone or cefotaxime plus ampicillin	Neonatal pneumonia or sepsis, ceftriaxone or cefotaxime plus ampicillin	For *S pneumoniae* see next column	Penicillin, ampicillin, or cefuroxime Cefotaxime or ceftriaxone Clindamycin Vancomycin until alternative susceptible agents are identified	Macrolides Cefuroxime plus macrolides Macrolides plus cefotaxime or ceftriaxone or clindamycin Vancomycin

Summary

Upper and lower airway infections are common in pediatrics and are usually diagnosed clinically based on the history, physical examination, and specific epidemiologic characteristics. Changes in pneumococcal resistance and immunization practices with pneumococcal and influenza vaccines will continue to change the incidence rate and causative findings of pneumonia. The treatment of airway infections is always supportive, but specific management strategies for certain pathogens, including the selection of antibiotics, bronchodilators, steroids, and inpatient or outpatient disposition, depend on the disease, the age, and the clinical characteristics of the host.

References

[1] Baker MD, Ruddy RM. Pulmonary emergencies. In: Ludwig S, editor. Textbook of pediatric emergency medicine. Philadelphia: Lippincott Williams & Wilkins; 2000. p. 1067–86.

[2] Bisno AL, Gerber MA, Gwaltney Jr JM, et al. Practice guidelines for the diagnosis and management of group A streptococcal pharyngitis. Clin Infect Dis 2002;35(2):113–25.

[3] McIsaac WJ, White D, Tannenbaum D, et al. A clinical score to reduce unnecessary antibiotic use in patients with sore throat. CMAJ 1998;158(1):75–83.

[4] Esposito S, Blasi F, Bosis S, et al. Aetiology of acute pharyngitis: the role of atypical bacteria. J Med Microbiol 2004;53(Pt 7):645–51.

[5] Chi H, Chiu NC, Li WC, et al. Etiology of acute pharyngitis in children: is antibiotic therapy needed? J Microbiol Immunol Infect 2003;36(1):26–30.

[6] Pickering LK. Red book: 2003 report of the Committee on Infectious Diseases. 26th edition. Elk Grove Village (IL): American Academy of Pediatrics; 2003.

[7] Hossain P, Kostiala A, Lyytikainen O, et al. Clinical features of district hospital paediatric patients with pharyngeal group A streptococci. Scand J Infect Dis 2003;35(1):77–9.

[8] Komaroff AL, Pass TM, Aronson MD, et al. The prediction of streptococcal pharyngitis in adults. J Gen Intern Med 1986;1(1):1–7.

[9] Centor RM, Witherspoon JM, Dalton HP, et al. The diagnosis of strep throat in adults in the emergency room. Med Decis Making 1981;1(3):239–46.

[10] Attia MW, Zaoutis T, Klein JD, et al. Performance of a predictive model for streptococcal pharyngitis in children. Arch Pediatr Adolesc Med 2001;155(6):687–91.

[11] McIsaac WJ, Kellner JD, Aufricht P, et al. Empirical validation of guidelines for the management of pharyngitis in children and adults. JAMA 2004;291(13):1587–95.

[12] Hall MC, Kieke B, Gonzales R, et al. Spectrum bias of a rapid antigen detection test for group A beta-hemolytic streptococcal pharyngitis in a pediatric population. Pediatrics 2004;114(1): 182–6.

[13] Dimatteo LA, Lowenstein SR, Brimhall B, et al. The relationship between the clinical features of pharyngitis and the sensitivity of a rapid antigen test: evidence of spectrum bias. Ann Emerg Med 2001;38(6):648–52.

[14] Dagnelie CF, Bartelink ML, van der Graaf Y, et al. Towards a better diagnosis of throat infections (with group A beta-haemolytic streptococcus) in general practice. Br J Gen Pract 1998;48(427):959–62.

[15] Gerber MA, Shulman ST. Rapid diagnosis of pharyngitis caused by group A streptococci. Clin Microbiol Rev 2004;17(3):571–80.

[16] Cohen R. Defining the optimum treatment regimen for azithromycin in acute tonsillopharyngitis. Pediatr Infect Dis J 2004;23(2 Suppl):S129–34.

[17] Ezike EN, Rongkavilit C, Fairfax MR, et al. Effect of using 2 throat swabs vs 1 throat swab on detection of group A streptococcus by a rapid antigen detection test. Arch Pediatr Adolesc Med 2005;159(5):486–90.

[18] Sun J, Keh-Gong W, Hwang B. Evaluation of the etiologic agents for acute suppurative tonsillitis in children. Zhonghua Yi Xue Za Zhi 2002;65(5):212–7.

[19] Shulman ST, Gerber MA. So what's wrong with penicillin for strep throat? Pediatrics 2004; 113(6):1816–9.

[20] Shvartzman P, Tabenkin H, Rosentzwaig A, et al. Treatment of streptococcal pharyngitis with amoxycillin once a day. BMJ 1993;306(6886):1170–2.

[21] Feder Jr HM, Gerber MA, Randolph MF, et al. Once-daily therapy for streptococcal pharyngitis with amoxicillin. Pediatrics 1999;103(1):47–51.

[22] Schaad UB, Kellerhals P, Altwegg M. Azithromycin versus penicillin V for treatment of acute group A streptococcal pharyngitis. Pediatr Infect Dis J 2002;21(4):304–8.

[23] Cohen R, Reinert P, De La Rocque F, et al. Comparison of two dosages of azithromycin for three days versus penicillin V for ten days in acute group A streptococcal tonsillopharyngitis. Pediatr Infect Dis J 2002;21(4):297–303.

[24] Syrogiannopoulos GA, Bozdogan B, Grivea IN, et al. Two dosages of clarithromycin for five days, amoxicillin/clavulanate for five days or penicillin V for ten days in acute group A streptococcal tonsillopharyngitis. Pediatr Infect Dis J 2004;23(9):857–65.

[25] Lazarevic G, Laban-Nestorovic S, Jovanovic M, et al. [Erythromycin-resistant *Streptococcus pyogenes*]. Srp Arh Celok Lek 2004;132(Suppl 1):S42–4.

[26] Martin JM, Green M, Barbadora KA, et al. Erythromycin-resistant group A streptococci in schoolchildren in Pittsburgh. N Engl J Med 2002;346(16):1200–6.

[27] Bertin L, d'Athis PG, Lasfargues G, et al. Randomized, double-blind, multicenter, controlled trial of ibuprofen versus acetaminophen (paracetamol) and placebo for treatment of symptoms of tonsillitis and pharyngitis in children. J Pediatr 1991;119(5):811–4.

[28] Olympia RP, Khine H, Avner JR. Effectiveness of oral dexamethasone in the treatment of moderate to severe pharyngitis in children. Arch Pediatr Adolesc Med 2005;159(3):278–82.

[29] Denny F, Murphy T, Clyde Jr W, et al. Croup: an 11-year study in a pediatric practice. Pediatrics 1983;71(6):871–6.

[30] Ausejo M, Saenz A, Pham B, et al. The effectiveness of glucocorticoids in treating croup: meta-analysis. BMJ 1999;319(7210):595–600.

[31] Segal AO, Crighton EJ, Moineddin R, et al. Croup hospitalizations in Ontario: a 14-year time-series analysis. Pediatrics 2005;116(1):51–5.

[32] Cummings CW. Otolaryngology: head & neck surgery. 4th edition. St. Louis: Mosby; 2005.

[33] Fogel JM, Berg IJ, Gerber MA, et al. Racemic epinephrine in the treatment of croup: nebulization alone versus nebulization with intermittent positive pressure breathing. J Pediatr 1982; 101(6):1028–31.

[34] Westley CR, Cotton EK, Brooks JG. Nebulized racemic epinephrine by IPPB for the treatment of croup: a double-blind study. Am J Dis Child 1978;132(5):484–7.

[35] Kuusela AL, Vesikari T. A randomized double-blind, placebo-controlled trial of dexamethasone and racemic epinephrine in the treatment of croup. Acta Paediatr Scand 1988;77(1):99–104.

[36] Bjornson CL, Klassen TP, Williamson J, et al. A randomized trial of a single dose of oral dexamethasone for mild croup. N Engl J Med 2004;351(13):1306–13.

[37] Geelhoed GC. Budesonide offers no advantage when added to oral dexamethasone in the treatment of croup. Pediatr Emerg Care 2005;21(6):359–60.

[38] Kelley PB, Simon JE. Racemic epinephrine use in croup and disposition. Am J Emerg Med 1992;10(3):181–3.

[39] Ledwith CA, Shea LM, Mauro RD. Safety and efficacy of nebulized racemic epinephrine in conjunction with oral dexamethasone and mist in the outpatient treatment of croup. Ann Emerg Med 1995;25(3):331–7.

[40] Kucera CM, Silverstein MD, Jacobson RM, et al. Epiglottitis in adults and children in Olmsted County, Minnesota, 1976 through 1990. Mayo Clin Proc 1996;71(12):1155–61.

[41] Solomon PWM, Irish JC, Gullane PJ. Adult epiglottitis: the Toronto Hospital experience. J Otolaryngol 1998;27(6):332–6.

[42] Rothrock G, Reingold A, Alexopoulos N. *Haemophilus influenzae* invasive disease among children aged < 5 years: California, 1990–1996. MMWR Morb Mortal Wkly Rep 1998;47(35): 737–40.

[43] Midwinter KI, Hodgson D, Yardley M. Paediatric epiglottitis: the influence of the *Haemophilus influenzae* b vaccine, a ten-year review in the Sheffield region. Clin Otolaryngol 1999;24(5): 447–8.

[44] Garpenholt OHS, Fredlund H, Bodin L, et al. Epiglottitis in Sweden before and after introduction of vaccination against *Haemophilus influenzae* type b. Pediatr Infect Dis J 1999; 18(6):490–3.

[45] Madore DV. Impact of immunization on *Haemophilus influenzae* type b disease. Infect Agents Dis 1996;5(1):8–20.

[46] Gonzalez Valdepena HWE, Rose E, Ungkanont K, et al. Epiglottitis and *Haemophilus influenzae* immunization: the Pittsburgh experience: a five-year review. Pediatrics 1995;96(3 Pt 1): 424–7.

[47] Alho OP, Jokinen K, Pirila T, et al. Acute epiglottitis and infant conjugate *Haemophilus influenzae* type b vaccination in northern Finland. Arch Otolaryngol Head Neck Surg 1995; 121(8):898–902.

[48] Shah RK, Roberson DW, Jones DT. Epiglottitis in the *Haemophilus influenzae* type B vaccine era: changing trends. Laryngoscope 2004;114(3):557–60.

[49] Mayo-Smith MF, Spinale JW, Donskey CJ, et al. Acute epiglottitis: an 18-year experience in Rhode Island. Chest 1995;108(6):1640–7.

[50] Berger G, Landau T, Berger S, et al. The rising incidence of adult acute epiglottitis and epiglottic abscess. Am J Otolaryngol 2003;24(6):374–83.

[51] McEwan J, Giridharan W, Clarke RW, et al. Paediatric acute epiglottitis: not a disappearing entity. Int J Pediatr Otorhinolaryngol 2003;67(4):317–21.

[52] Wagle A, Jones RM. Acute epiglottitis despite vaccination with *Haemophilus influenzae* type B vaccine. Paediatr Anaesth 1999;9(6):549–50.

[53] Berg S, Trollfors B, Nylen O, et al. Incidence, aetiology, and prognosis of acute epiglottitis in children and adults in Sweden. Scand J Infect Dis 1996;28(3):261–4.

[54] Brook I. Microbiology and management of peritonsillar, retropharyngeal, and parapharyngeal abscesses. J Oral Maxillofac Surg 2004;62(12):1545–50.

[55] Powderly C. Infectious diseases. New York: Elsevier; 2004. p. 460.

[56] Philpott CM, Selvadurai D, Banerjee AR. Paediatric retropharyngeal abscess. J Laryngol Otol 2004;118(12):919–26.

[57] Daya H, Lo S, Papsin BC, et al. Retropharyngeal and parapharyngeal infections in children: the Toronto experience. Int J Pediatr Otorhinolaryngol 2005;69(1):81–6.

[58] Craig FW, Schunk JE. Retropharyngeal abscess in children: clinical presentation, utility of imaging, and current management. Pediatrics 2003;111(6 Pt 1):1394–8.

[59] Dawes LC, Bova R, Carter P. Retropharyngeal abscess in children. ANZ J Surg 2002;72(6): 417–20.

[60] Liu CH, Lin CD, Cheng YK, et al. Deep neck infection in children. Acta Paediatr Taiwan 2004; 45(5):265–8.

[61] Haug RH, Wible RT, Lieberman J. Measurement standards for the prevertebral region in the lateral soft-tissue radiograph of the neck. J Oral Maxillofac Surg 1991;49(11):1149–51.

[62] Al-Sabah B, Bin Salleen H, Hagr A, et al. Retropharyngeal abscess in children: 10-year study. J Otolaryngol 2004;33(6):352–5.

[63] Nagy M, Pizzuto M, Backstrom J, et al. Deep neck infections in children: a new approach to diagnosis and treatment. Laryngoscope 1997;107(12 Pt 1):1627–34.

[64] Kirse DJ, Roberson DW. Surgical management of retropharyngeal space infections in children. Laryngoscope 2001;111(8):1413–22.

[65] Ben-Ami T, Yousefzadeh DK, Aramburo MJ. Pre-suppurative phase of retropharyngeal infec-

tion: contribution of ultrasonography in the diagnosis and treatment. Pediatr Radiol 1990;21(1): 23–6.

[66] Chao HC, Chiu CH, Lin SJ, et al. Colour Doppler ultrasonography of retropharyngeal abscess. J Otolaryngol 1999;28(3):138–41.

[67] Glasier CM, Stark JE, Jacobs RF, et al. CT and ultrasound imaging of retropharyngeal abscesses in children. AJNR Am J Neuroradiol 1992;13(4):1191–5.

[68] Dufour X, Gohler C, Bedier A, et al. [Retropharyngeal and lateral pharyngeal abscesses in children]. Ann Otolaryngol Chir Cervicofac 2004;121(6):327–33.

[69] Ong YK, Goh YH, Lee YL. Peritonsillar infections: local experience. Singapore Med J 2004; 45(3):105–9.

[70] Szuhay G, Tewfik TL. Peritonsillar abscess or cellulitis? a clinical comparative paediatric study. J Otolaryngol 1998;27(4):206–12.

[71] Friedman NR, Mitchell RB, Pereira KD, et al. Peritonsillar abscess in early childhood: presentation and management. Arch Otolaryngol Head Neck Surg 1997;123(6):630–2.

[72] Miziara ID, Koishi HU, Zonato AI, et al. The use of ultrasound evaluation in the diagnosis of peritonsillar abscess. Rev Laryngol Otol Rhinol (Bord) 2001;122(3):201–3.

[73] Suskind DL, Park J, Piccirillo JF, et al. Conscious sedation: a new approach for peritonsillar abscess drainage in the pediatric population. Arch Otolaryngol Head Neck Surg 1999;125(11): 1197–200.

[74] Bauer PW, Lieu JE, Suskind DL, et al. The safety of conscious sedation in peritonsillar abscess drainage. Arch Otolaryngol Head Neck Surg 2001;127(12):1477–80.

[75] Luhmann JD, Kennedy RM, McAllister JD, et al. Sedation for peritonsillar abscess drainage in the pediatric emergency department. Pediatr Emerg Care 2002;18(1):1–3.

[76] Ramirez S, Hild TG, Rudolph CN, et al. Increased diagnosis of Lemierre syndrome and other *Fusobacterium necrophorum* infections at a Children's Hospital. Pediatrics 2003; 112(5):E380.

[77] Matsuda A, Tanaka H, Kanaya T, et al. Peritonsillar abscess: a study of 724 cases in Japan. Ear Nose Throat J 2002;81(6):384–9.

[78] Williams A, Nagy M, Wingate J, et al. Lemierre syndrome: a complication of acute pharyngitis. Int J Pediatr Otorhinolaryngol 1998;45(1):51–7.

[79] Jokinen C, Heiskanen L, Juvonen H, et al. Incidence of community-acquired pneumonia in the population of four municipalities in eastern Finland. Am J Epidemiol 1993;137(9):977–88.

[80] Murphy TF, Henderson FW, Clyde Jr WA, et al. Pneumonia: an eleven-year study in a pediatric practice. Am J Epidemiol 1981;113(1):12–21.

[81] WHO Young Infants Study Group. Serious infections in young infants in developing countries: rationale for a multicenter study. Pediatr Infect Dis J 1999;18(10 Suppl):S4–7.

[82] Mulholland EK, Simoes EA, Costales MO, et al. Standardized diagnosis of pneumonia in developing countries. Pediatr Infect Dis J 1992;11(2):77–81.

[83] McCracken Jr GH. Diagnosis and management of pneumonia in children. Pediatr Infect Dis J 2000;19(9):924–8.

[84] Ngai P, Bye MR. Bronchiolitis. Pediatr Ann 2002;31(2):90–7.

[85] Simoes EA. Respiratory syncytial virus infection. Lancet 1999;354(9181):847–52.

[86] Weiner DJ. Respiratory tract infections in cystic fibrosis. Pediatr Ann 2002;31(2):116–23.

[87] Foy HM, Cooney MK, Allan I, et al. Rates of pneumonia during influenza epidemics in Seattle, 1964 to 1975. JAMA 1979;241(3):253–8.

[88] McConnochie KM, Hall CB, Barker WH. Lower respiratory tract illness in the first two years of life: epidemiologic patterns and costs in a suburban pediatric practice. Am J Public Health 1988;78(1):34–9.

[89] Selwyn BJ for the Coordinated Data Group of BOSTID Researchers. The epidemiology of acute respiratory tract infection in young children: comparison of findings from several developing countries. Rev Infect Dis 1990;12(Suppl 8):S870–88.

[90] Armengot M, Escribano A, Carda C, et al. Clinical and ultrastructural correlations in nasal mucociliary function observed in children with recurrent airways infections. Int J Pediatr Otorhinolaryngol 1995;32(2):143–51.

[91] Bauer ML, Figueroa-Colon R, et al. Chronic pulmonary aspiration in children. South Med J 1993;86(7):789–95.
[92] Shackelford PG, Polmar SH, Mayus JL, et al. Spectrum of IgG2 subclass deficiency in children with recurrent infections: prospective study. J Pediatr 1986;108(5 Pt 1):647–53.
[93] Kravitz RM. Congenital malformations of the lung. Pediatr Clin North Am 1994;41(3):453–72.
[94] Mansbach JM, Emond JA, Camargo Jr CA. Bronchiolitis in US emergency departments 1992 to 2000: epidemiology and practice variation. Pediatr Emerg Care 2005;21(4):242–7.
[95] Ruuskanen O, Mertsola J. Childhood community-acquired pneumonia. Semin Respir Infect 1999;14(2):163–72.
[96] Juven T, Mertsola J, Waris M, et al. Etiology of community-acquired pneumonia in 254 hospitalized children. Pediatr Infect Dis J 2000;19(4):293–8.
[97] Lichenstein R, Suggs AH, Campbell J. Pediatric pneumonia. Emerg Med Clin North Am 2003; 21(2):437–51.
[98] Heiskanen-Kosma T, Korppi M, Jokinen C, et al. Etiology of childhood pneumonia: serologic results of a prospective, population-based study. Pediatr Infect Dis J 1998;17(11):986–91.
[99] Wubbel L, Muniz L, Ahmed A, et al. Etiology and treatment of community-acquired pneumonia in ambulatory children. Pediatr Infect Dis J 1999;18(2):98–104.
[100] Harris JA, Kolokathis A, Campbell M, et al. Safety and efficacy of azithromycin in the treatment of community-acquired pneumonia in children. Pediatr Infect Dis J 1998;17(10): 865–71.
[101] Block S, Hedrick J, Hammerschlag MR, et al. Mycoplasma pneumoniae and Chlamydia pneumoniae in pediatric community-acquired pneumonia: comparative efficacy and safety of clarithromycin vs. erythromycin ethylsuccinate. Pediatr Infect Dis J 1995;14(6):471–7.
[102] McIntosh K. Community-acquired pneumonia in children. N Engl J Med 2002;346(6):429–37.
[103] Tan TQ, Mason Jr EO, Barson WJ, et al. Clinical characteristics and outcome of children with pneumonia attributable to penicillin-susceptible and penicillin-nonsusceptible Streptococcus pneumoniae. Pediatrics 1998;102(6):1369–75.
[104] Whitney CG, Farley MM, Hadler J, et al. Increasing prevalence of multidrug-resistant Streptococcus pneumoniae in the United States. N Engl J Med 2000;343(26):1917–24.
[105] Levine MM, Lagos R, Levine OS, et al. Epidemiology of invasive pneumococcal infections in infants and young children in Metropolitan Santiago, Chile, a newly industrializing country. Pediatr Infect Dis J 1998;17(4):287–93.
[106] American Academy of Pediatrics Committee on Infectious Diseases. Therapy for children with invasive pneumococcal infections. Pediatrics 1997;99(2):289–99.
[107] McCracken Jr GH. Etiology and treatment of pneumonia. Pediatr Infect Dis J 2000;19(4): 373–7.
[108] Kaplan SL, Mason Jr EO. Mechanisms of pneumococcal antibiotic resistance and treatment of pneumococcal infections in 2002. Pediatr Ann 2002;31(4):250–60.
[109] Dawson KP, Long A, Kennedy J, et al. The chest radiograph in acute bronchiolitis. J Paediatr Child Health 1990;26(4):209–11.
[110] Lichenstein R, King Jr JC, Lovchik J, et al. Respiratory viral infections in hospitalized children: implications for infection control. South Med J 2002;95(9):1022–5.
[111] Shaw KN, Bell LM, Sherman NH. Outpatient assessment of infants with bronchiolitis. Am J Dis Child 1991;145(2):151–5.
[112] Klassen TP. Recent advances in the treatment of bronchiolitis and laryngitis. Pediatr Clin North Am 1997;44(1):249–61.
[113] Law BJ, Wang EE, MacDonald N, et al. Does ribavirin impact on the hospital course of children with respiratory syncytial virus (RSV) infection? an analysis using the pediatric investigators collaborative network on infections in Canada (PICNIC) RSV database. Pediatrics 1997;99(3):E7.
[114] Chipps BE, Sullivan WF, Portnoy JM. Alpha-2A-interferon for treatment of bronchiolitis caused by respiratory syncytial virus. Pediatr Infect Dis J 1993;12(8):653–8.
[115] Bisgaard H. A randomized trial of montelukast in respiratory syncytial virus postbronchiolitis. Am J Respir Crit Care Med 2003;167(3):379–83.

[116] Flores G, Horwitz RI. Efficacy of beta2-agonists in bronchiolitis: a reappraisal and meta-analysis. Pediatrics 1997;100(2 Pt 1):233–9.

[117] Bertrand P, Aranibar H, Castro E, et al. Efficacy of nebulized epinephrine versus salbutamol in hospitalized infants with bronchiolitis. Pediatr Pulmonol 2001;31(4):284–8.

[118] Garrison MM, Christakis DA, Harvey E, et al. Systemic corticosteroids in infant bronchiolitis: a meta-analysis. Pediatrics 2000;105(4):E44.

[119] Kellner JD, Ohlsson A, Gadomski AM, et al. Bronchodilators for bronchiolitis. Cochrane Database Syst Rev 2000;2:CD001266.

[120] Schweich PJ, Hurt TL, Walkley EI, et al. The use of nebulized albuterol in wheezing infants. Pediatr Emerg Care 1992;8(4):184–8.

[121] Schuh S, Canny G, Reisman JJ, et al. Nebulized albuterol in acute bronchiolitis. J Pediatr 1990; 117(4):633–7.

[122] Reijonen T, Korppi M, Pitkakangas S, et al. The clinical efficacy of nebulized racemic epinephrine and albuterol in acute bronchiolitis. Arch Pediatr Adolesc Med 1995;149(6):686–92.

[123] Sanchez I, De Koster J, Powell RE, et al. Effect of racemic epinephrine and salbutamol on clinical score and pulmonary mechanics in infants with bronchiolitis. J Pediatr 1993;122(1): 145–51.

[124] Schuh S, Johnson D, Canny G, et al. Efficacy of adding nebulized ipratropium bromide to nebulized albuterol therapy in acute bronchiolitis. Pediatrics 1992;90(6):920–3.

[125] Roosevelt G, Sheehan K, Grupp-Phelan J, et al. Dexamethasone in bronchiolitis: a randomised controlled trial. Lancet 1996;348(9023):292–5.

[126] Klassen TP, Sutcliffe T, Watters LK, et al. Dexamethasone in salbutamol-treated inpatients with acute bronchiolitis: a randomized, controlled trial. J Pediatr 1997;130(2):191–6.

[127] Richter H, Seddon P. Early nebulized budesonide in the treatment of bronchiolitis and the prevention of postbronchiolitic wheezing. J Pediatr 1998;132(5):849–53.

[128] Schuh S, Coates AL, Binnie R, et al. Efficacy of oral dexamethasone in outpatients with acute bronchiolitis. J Pediatr 2002;140(1):27–32.

[129] van Woensel JB, Wolfs TF, van Aalderen WM, et al. Randomised double blind placebo controlled trial of prednisolone in children admitted to hospital with respiratory syncytial virus bronchiolitis. Thorax 1997;52(7):634–7.

[130] Plint AC, Johnson DW, Wiebe N, et al. Practice variation among pediatric emergency departments in the treatment of bronchiolitis. Acad Emerg Med 2004;11(4):353–60.

[131] Johnson DW, Adair C, Brant R, et al. Differences in admission rates of children with bronchiolitis by pediatric and general emergency departments. Pediatrics 2002;110(4):E49.

[132] Mallory MD, Shay DK, Garrett J, et al. Bronchiolitis management preferences and the influence of pulse oximetry and respiratory rate on the decision to admit. Pediatrics 2003;111(1):E45–51.

[133] Hindiyeh M, Carroll KC. Laboratory diagnosis of atypical pneumonia. Semin Respir Infect 2000;15(2):101–13.

[134] Falguera M, Sacristan O, Nogues A, et al. Nonsevere community-acquired pneumonia: correlation between cause and severity or comorbidity. Arch Intern Med 2001;161(15):1866–72.

[135] Fleisher GR, Ludwig S. Textbook of pediatric emergency medicine. 4th edition. Baltimore (MD): Williams & Wilkins; 2000.

[136] Michelow IC, Olsen K, Lozano J, et al. Epidemiology and clinical characteristics of community-acquired pneumonia in hospitalized children. Pediatrics 2004;113(4):701–7.

[137] Graham SM, Mtitimila EI, Kamanga HS, et al. Clinical presentation and outcome of Pneumocystis carinii pneumonia in Malawian children. Lancet 2000;355(9201):369–73.

[138] Dowell SF, Kupronis BA, Zell ER, et al. Mortality from pneumonia in children in the United States, 1939 through 1996. N Engl J Med 2000;342(19):1399–407.

[139] Marrie TJ, Lau CY, Wheeler SL, et al for the Community-Acquired Pneumonia Intervention Trial Assessing Levofloxacin (CAPITAL) Study Investigators. A controlled trial of a critical pathway for treatment of community-acquired pneumonia. JAMA 2000;283(6):749–55.

[140] Committee on Infectious Diseases. Red book 2000: report of the Committee on Infectious Diseases. In: Pickering L, editor. Elk Grove Village (IL): American Academy of Pediatrics; 2000. p. 208–12.

[141] Heininger U, Klich K, Stehr K, et al. Clinical findings in *Bordetella pertussis* infections: results of a prospective multicenter surveillance study. Pediatrics 1997;100(6):E10.

[142] Committee on Infectious Diseases. Red book 2000: report of the Committee on Infectious Diseases. In: Pickering L, editor. 25th edition. Elk Grove Village (IL): American Academy of Pediatrics; 2000. p. 435–48.

[143] Mink CA, Sirota NM, Nugent S. Outbreak of pertussis in a fully immunized adolescent and adult population. Arch Pediatr Adolesc Med 1994;148(2):153–7.

[144] Pertussis: United States, 1997–2000. MMWR Morb Mortal Wkly Rep 2002;51(4):73–6.

[145] Guris D, Strebel PM, Bardenheier B, et al. Changing epidemiology of pertussis in the United States: increasing reported incidence among adolescents and adults, 1990–1996. Clin Infect Dis 1999;28(6):1230–7.

[146] Mikelova LK, Halperin SA, Scheifele D, et al. Predictors of death in infants hospitalized with pertussis: a case-control study of 16 pertussis deaths in Canada. J Pediatr 2003;143(5): 576–81.

[147] Tozzi AE, Rava L, Ciofi degli Atti ML, et al. Clinical presentation of pertussis in unvaccinated and vaccinated children in the first six years of life. Pediatrics 2003;112(5):1069–75.

[148] Cherry JD, Heininger U. Pertussis and other *bordetella* infections. In: Textbook of pediatric infectious diseases. Philadelphia: WB Saunders; 2004.

[149] Langley JM, Halperin SA, Boucher FD, et al. Azithromycin is as effective as and better tolerated than erythromycin estolate for the treatment of pertussis. Pediatrics 2004;114(1):E96–101.

[150] Toikka P, Virkki R, Mertsola J, et al. Bacteremic pneumococcal pneumonia in children. Clin Infect Dis 1999;29(3):568–72.

[151] Meeker DP, Longworth DL. Community-acquired pneumonia: an update. Cleve Clin J Med 1996;63(1):16–30.

[152] Musher DM, Spindel SJ. Community-acquired pneumonia. Curr Clin Top Infect Dis 1996;16: 102–24.

[153] Jadavji T, Law B, Lebel MH, et al. A practical guide for the diagnosis and treatment of pediatric pneumonia. CMAJ 1997;156(5):S703–11.

[154] Rothrock SG, Green SM, Fanelli JM, et al. Do published guidelines predict pneumonia in children presenting to an urban ED? Pediatr Emerg Care 2001;17(4):240–3.

[155] Lynch T, Platt R, Gouin S, et al. Can we predict which children with clinically suspected pneumonia will have the presence of focal infiltrates on chest radiographs? Pediatrics 2004; 113(3 Pt 1):E186–9.

[156] Courtoy I, Lande AE, Turner RB. Accuracy of radiographic differentiation of bacterial from nonbacterial pneumonia. Clin Pediatr (Phila) 1989;28(6):261–4.

[157] McCarthy PL, Spiesel SZ, Stashwick CA, et al. Radiographic findings and etiologic diagnosis in ambulatory childhood pneumonias. Clin Pediatr (Phila) 1981;20(11):686–91.

[158] Korppi M, Kiekara O, Heiskanen-Kosma T, et al. Comparison of radiological findings and microbial aetiology of childhood pneumonia. Acta Paediatr 1993;82(4):360–3.

[159] Markowitz RI, Ruchelli E. Pneumonia in infants and children: radiological-pathological correlation. Semin Roentgenol 1998;33(2):151–62.

[160] Condon VR. Pneumonia in children. J Thorac Imaging 1991;6(3):31–44.

[161] Wildin SR, Chonmaitree T, Swischuk LE. Roentgenographic features of common pediatric viral respiratory tract infections. Am J Dis Child 1988;142(1):43–6.

[162] Radkowski MA, Kranzler JK, Beem MO, et al. *Chlamydia* pneumonia in infants: radiography in 125 cases. AJR Am J Roentgenol 1981;137(4):703–6.

[163] Guckel C, Benz-Bohm G, Widemann B. Mycoplasmal pneumonias in childhood: roentgen features, differential diagnosis and review of literature. Pediatr Radiol 1989;19(8):499–503.

[164] Neu N, Saiman L, San Gabriel P, et al. Diagnosis of pediatric tuberculosis in the modern era. Pediatr Infect Dis J 1999;18(2):122–6.

[165] Nelson JD. Community-acquired pneumonia in children: guidelines for treatment. Pediatr Infect Dis J 2000;19(3):251–3.

[166] Korppi M, Kroger L. C-reactive protein in viral and bacterial respiratory infection in children. Scand J Infect Dis 1993;25(2):207–13.

[167] Ponka A, Sarna S. Differential diagnosis of viral, mycoplasmal and bacteraemic pneumococcal pneumonias on admission to hospital. Eur J Respir Dis 1983;64(5):360–8.

[168] Korppi M, Kroger L, Laitinen M. White blood cell and differential counts in acute respiratory viral and bacterial infections in children. Scand J Infect Dis 1993;25(4):435–40.

[169] Michelow IC, Lozano J, Olsen K, et al. Diagnosis of *Streptococcus pneumoniae* lower respiratory infection in hospitalized children by culture, polymerase chain reaction, serological testing, and urinary antigen detection. Clin Infect Dis 2002;34(1):E1–11.

[170] Cohen GJ. Management of infections of the lower respiratory tract in children. Pediatr Infect Dis J 1987;6(3):317–23.

[171] Smyth A, Carty H, Hart CA. Clinical predictors of hypoxaemia in children with pneumonia. Ann Trop Paediatr 1998;18(1):31–40.

[172] Madico G, Gilman RH, Jabra A, et al. The role of pulse oximetry: its use as an indicator of severe respiratory disease in Peruvian children living at sea level. Arch Pediatr Adolesc Med 1995;149(11):1259–63.

[173] Lozano JM, Steinhoff M, Ruiz JG, et al. Clinical predictors of acute radiological pneumonia and hypoxaemia at high altitude. Arch Dis Child 1994;71(4):323–7.

[174] Campbell JD, Nataro JP. Pleural empyema. Pediatr Infect Dis J 1999;18(8):725–6.

[175] Mace SE. Pediatric observation medicine. Emerg Med Clin North Am 2001;1(1):239–54.

ELSEVIER
SAUNDERS

PEDIATRIC CLINICS
OF NORTH AMERICA

Pediatr Clin N Am 53 (2006) 243–256

Pediatric Blunt Abdominal Trauma

Stephen Wegner, MD[a],*, James E. Colletti, MD[b],
Donald Van Wie, DO[c]

[a]Emergency Medical Services, Blackfeet Community Hospital, PO Box 760, Browning,
MT 59417, USA
[b]Emergency Medicine Regions Hospital, 640 Jackson Street, St. Paul, MN 55101-2502, USA
[c]Division of Emergency Medicine, Department of Surgery, Department of Pediatrics,
University of Maryland School of Medicine, 110 South Paca Street, Sixth Floor, Suite 200,
Baltimore, MD 21201, USA

Despite increased awareness and prevention efforts, trauma remains the number one cause of childhood death and disability [1]. According to the national pediatric trauma registry, each year approximately 1.5 million children are injured, resulting in 500,000 pediatric hospitalizations, 120,000 children with permanent disability, and 20,000 deaths. Although abdominal trauma is less common than isolated head injury, it is still a leading cause of morbidity and mortality in children. In certain scenarios, particularly in preverbal children or children with a decreased level of consciousness, identification of an abdominal injury can be challenging, and failure to detect these injuries initially can lead to preventable complications. Nationwide, injured children are cared for not only at dedicated pediatric trauma centers but also in emergency departments and clinics that may not routinely evaluate children for these injuries. All clinicians who care for children with potential blunt abdominal injuries should be aware of current concepts related to the diagnosis and treatment of pediatric blunt abdominal trauma.

In this article we discuss key issues to help clinicians efficiently and successfully evaluate and manage blunt pediatric abdominal trauma. We also briefly review select organ trauma, including trauma that involves liver, spleen, intestines, pancreas, and kidneys. Finally, we discuss some of the disposition issues,

---

* Corresponding author.
  E-mail address: Stephen.wegner@mail.ihs.gov (S. Wegner).

doi:10.1016/j.pcl.2006.02.002

including length of hospitalization and return to activity recommendations for children with intra-abdominal injuries (IAI).

Mechanism of injury

Consideration of the cause of blunt pediatric abdominal trauma has been a major decision point for pediatric trauma system activation and deciding how to evaluate a child for potential IAI. Motor vehicle collisions (without proper restraint and ejection from a vehicle), automobile versus pedestrian accidents, and falls are associated with the greatest increased risk of IAI [2–4]. Other mechanisms of concern that should prompt close evaluation for IAI include children in a motor vehicle collision wearing only lap belt restraints, automobile versus bicycle accident, all-terrain vehicle accidents, handlebar injuries from bicycles, and sports or nonaccidental trauma resulting in direct blows to the abdomen [2,5,6]. There is a case series involving two 5-year-old children who played "superman" (the children attempted to fly off a top dresser to a crib and instead of landing in the crib struck the railing of the crib with their abdomens), which resulted in IAI [6].

Several studies have outlined that abdomen-to-handlebar collisions are associated with a high risk of small bowel and pancreatic trauma [7,8]. This trauma can occur after seemingly harmless incidents, and direct impact on the handlebars may result in more severe injuries than flipping over them [8]. Childhood sports and recreational activities, although generally safe, can produce IAI. In a study of adolescents in western New York, Wan and colleagues [9] found that injuries occurred in 0.73% of sports participants; the organs injured in descending frequency were kidney, spleen, and liver. Of note, the authors found that sledding and snowboarding resulted in injuries more often than football. This finding was echoed by a Canadian report that found that snowboarding resulted in IAI six times more frequently than skiers [10].

Past medical history

Obtaining as much information as possible about a child's past medical history is always worthwhile even in the abbreviated trauma history and examination. Medical conditions that affect children's neurologic or developmental baseline are important to obtain from any sources available to the provider. A few examples that may make evaluation of a child more difficult include autism, cerebral palsy, or other medical conditions that result in mental or physical handicaps. Hemophilia is also of particular concern, and careful evaluation and management of children with this disease are warranted. Several reports in the literature cite the risk of delayed splenic rupture and massive bleeding from minor abdominal trauma in children who have hemophilia [11,12]. In addition to inherited bleeding disorders, any pediatric patient who is being anticoagulated or receiving antiplatelet therapy (eg, for acquired or congenital heart defects) should be considered to be at higher risk for bleeding and significant IAI. It is important to inquire about recent or concurrent Epstein-Barr virus infection (secondary to the risk of splenic injury from even minor abdominal trauma in children with splenomegaly from Epstein-Barr virus).

Physical examination

When discussing the importance of physical examination findings in a child with a potentially serious IAI, certain key concepts should be emphasized. First, an abdominal examination abnormality should be considered an indicator of IAI. Second, in addition to the abdominal examination, other associated comorbid injuries or factors predict abdominal injury. Third, despite the helpfulness of the first two factors, a negative examination and absence of comorbid injuries do not totally rule out an IAI.

Holmes and colleagues [2] performed a prospective observational study of 1095 children and determined abdominal tenderness to be predictive of IAI (odds ratio [OR] 5.8). The authors did not calculate positive predictive value or negative predictive value in the study, but the article's data indicate that they were 17%, and 93%, respectively. Cotton and colleagues [5] identified abdominal tenderness, ecchymosis, and abrasions as positive predictors of IAI (ORs were 40.7, 15.8 and 16.8, respectively). Isaacman et al [13] performed a retrospective review of 285 pediatric trauma patients classified as moderately injured (14 of the 285 were identified to have a significant IAI) and found that an abnormal physical examination plus an abnormal urinalysis (UA) to be a highly sensitive screen for IAI (sensitivity, specificity, positive predictive value, and negative predictive value were 100%, 64%, 13%, and 100%, respectively). Another study in 1997 looked specifically at small bowel injury and found that 94% of the time there was exam pathology and of the 13 CT scans that were performed on the patients with small bowel injury, only one was positive [14]. This evidence suggests that imaging is indicated in children with abnormal abdominal examinations.

Although this statement seems obvious, the more frequently encountered clinical scenario that may challenge the provider is when CT imaging should be obtained on children who have benign abdominal examinations but have a concerning medical history or mechanism. The first clue is to look at comorbid findings in a child with potential IAI, and the second is to look at select laboratory values.

Associated comorbid findings/injuries can help predict which children have abdominal injury. Two of these findings came from the 2004 Holmes study, the first of which was the presence of a femur fracture (OR 1.3) [2]. Although this finding only has a mild increased risk for IAI, given the seriousness of a missed IAI, the provider should consider strongly using the presence of a femur fracture in a child as a reason to obtain further diagnostic imaging. The second finding that can help predict IAI from the Holmes study is low systolic blood pressure with an OR for IAI of 4.8 [2]. This is not necessarily a surprise and does not have strong sensitive or specificity, but it does indicate another finding that, when present, may lead a clinician to consider abdominal CT imaging.

Another factor that has been correlated with IAI (or at least may mask a reliable physical examination that would make a clinician suspect IAI) is a decrease in mental status. The Holmes investigation identified a Glasgow Coma Score of less than 13 as a mild indicator of IAI with an OR of 1.7. This finding was enough for the authors to recommend obtaining CT imaging in patients with a Glasgow Coma Score less than 13 [2]. Another prospective study by Beaver and colleagues [15] revealed that in patients with a Glasgow Coma Score less than 10, 23% had significant IAI. A final point of consideration is that there is much concern about the reliability of abdominal examination in preverbal children. Although this age group is included in studies that addressed pediatric blunt abdominal trauma, preverbal children are underrepresented and not specifically substratified. The provider must consider the mechanism of trauma in assessing risk of injury. Because the risk of IAI varies greatly with each given mechanism of trauma in the preverbal age group, the provider should err on the side of caution in considering whether to obtain further laboratory testing or radiographic imaging.

Laboratory testing

After the history and physical examination, the next step in evaluating pediatric patients with potential IAI is what laboratory test should be obtained. In a hypotensive child who is unresponsive to isotonic fluid boluses, the type and cross is the most important test to order. Most children with abdominal injuries are not hypotensive, however, and there are two reasons for performing laboratory testing. The first reason is to treat a potentially unstable patient immediately. The second reason is to screen stable children for a possible IAI. When considering which laboratory tests to order, it is important that the clinician avoid routine "trauma panel" testing in pediatric trauma patients. One example to support this practice can be demonstrated in a retrospective review by Keller and colleagues [16], in which 77% of patients in their trauma center had a type and cross performed, yet only 3.8% of the patients actually received blood.

The second reason to order laboratory tests is to help predict which children may have IAI. The most useful laboratory tests for this purpose include the complete blood count (CBC), liver function tests (LFTs), and UA. Also studied in the literature are amylase, lipase, coagulation studies, and general chemistries. Often these tests are part of standard trauma panels but not all are useful.

The CBC is a ubiquitous test drawn in almost every clinical situation [16]. The use of this test in pediatric trauma is mainly relegated to looking at the hemoglobin/hematocrit of patients. Initial serum values vary widely. In the study by Holmes and colleagues [2], an initial hematocrit of less than 30 had an OR of 2.6 for IAI. In 1993, however, Isaacman and colleagues [13] found that serial hematocrit used to detect IAI was a poor test. The greatest use for the hemoglobin and hematocrit is to follow serial values in known solid organ injuries. An initial hemoglobin and hematocrit are recommended in the evaluation of patients with pediatric abdominal trauma, but they should not be used to decide whether to perform an additional imaging study.

Coagulation studies (eg, prothrombin time, international normalized ratio, partial thromboplastin time) are sometimes drawn. It is well documented in the literature that a closed head injury leads to coagulation abnormalities [16,17]. When caring for pediatric patients who have blunt abdominal trauma without concomitant head injury or other premorbid conditions, no studies show that routine coagulation studies are beneficial.

Another routine trauma panel test often ordered is liver transaminases. The rationale is that liver enzyme release (alanine aminotransferase [AST] or aspartate aminotransferase [ALT]) is a marker for liver or other solid organ injury. Isaacman and colleagues [13] combined physical examination with a positive transaminase screen (AST or ALT >130) and claimed a 100% sensitive with 100% negative predictive value. Keller and colleagues [16,17] obtained a panel of laboratory tests (CBC, chemistry, coagulation panel, and UA) on 240 injured children younger than age 16. The authors concluded that routine laboratory data are of limited value in the management of injured children [16,18,19]. Puranik and colleagues [20] performed a chart review in 44 hemodynamically stable children with blunt abdominal trauma who had undergone abdominal CT. The authors compared AST and ALT levels in children with and without CT evidence of liver injury. They found an association between AST and ALT levels and CT evidence of liver injury. (Sensitivity and specificity of elevated liver enzyme levels were 92.2% and 100%, respectively, for predicting liver injury.) The authors concluded that an abdominal CT is indicated in pediatric blunt abdominal trauma when the AST is >400 or ALT >250. There was no significant evidence that LFTs were able to predict injuries that required an intervention, however [20].

In 2004, Cotton and colleagues [5] reported in a retrospective review that an elevated AST >131 plus abdominal findings had a sensitivity of 100% for detecting IAI. They also noted in patients without any abdominal tenderness that an ALT >101 had a sensitivity of 100% for detecting IAI [5]. A prospective observation series by Holmes and colleagues [2] enrolled 1095 children (107 had IAI) younger than age 16 who sustained blunt trauma. The authors identified six findings associated with an IAI (low systolic blood pressure, abdominal tenderness, femur fracture, elevated LFTs, UA with >5 red blood cells per high-powered field [hpf], initial hematocrit <30%). An ALT >125 or an AST >200 was determined to have an OR of 17.4; 95% CI 9.4 to 32.1 (54% of patients with elevated liver transaminases had an IAI) [2]. They concluded that laboratory testing contributes significantly to the identification of children with IAI after blunt trauma. Based on the evidence, it is reasonable to include an AST and ALT as part of an evaluation in a child with history of blunt abdominal trauma and an equivocal examination.

The UA is often routinely obtained in children with abdominal trauma. Microscopic hematuria has been defined differently by different authors as more than 5 red blood cells (RBC)/hpf, more than 20 RBC/hpf, or more than 50 RBC/hpf [2,13,21,22]. Gross hematuria is defined as hematuria visible to the clinician [2]. Gross and microscopic hematuria has been associated with the presence of an IAI in the blunt trauma pediatric patient [2,23]. The use of microscopic hematuria in evaluation of pediatric blunt abdominal is controversial, however [2,13,22–24].

Stein and colleagues [23] retrospectively evaluated the abdominal CT scans of 412 children, 48 of whom had CT documented renal injuries (25 of the 48 had significant renal injuries). All of the children with significant renal injuries presented with hematuria. Sixty-eight percent (17 of 25) had microscopic hematuria, and 32% (8 of 25) had gross hematuria. The authors concluded that any child who presents with blunt abdominal trauma and any evidence of hematuria should undergo abdominal and pelvic CT.

Stalker and colleagues [22] performed a retrospective chart review of 256 children with blunt abdominal trauma. One hundred six children presented with hematuria, and 35 had a renal injury diagnosed by abdominal CT. The authors commented that normotensive children with less than 50 RBC/hpf were not found to have a significant renal injury.

Taylor and colleagues [24] evaluated 378 children with blunt trauma. Hematuria was present in 256 children, of whom 168 had microscopic hematuria $\geq$10 RBC/hpf. In cases of asymptomatic hematuria, the risk of abdominal injury was negligible (0 of 41 patients). The authors concluded that asymptomatic hematuria is a low-yield indication for obtaining an abdominal CT in the pediatric patient who has blunt abdominal trauma.

Holmes and colleagues [2] performed a prospective analysis of laboratory testing in pediatric blunt abdominal trauma in which they considered microscopic hematuria to be >5 RBC/hpf. The authors concluded that hematuria more than 5 RBC/hpf is an important predictor of IAI in pediatric blunt trauma patients (OR of 4.8). In their recursive portioning analysis it was a more proximal node than abdominal tenderness. This is also echoed by an earlier investigation by Isaacman and colleagues [13] in which a negative UA and a normal physical examination had a negative predictive value of 100%. An investigation by Cotton and colleagues [5] with a similar statistical analysis of a smaller number of patients failed to discover a use for UA in pediatric blunt trauma patients. This debate still flourishes, especially in patients who are otherwise healthy without tenderness. Providers are cautioned in an area in which there is no definitive study to categorize patients according to mechanism of injury in conjunction with physical examination.

Table 1
Summary of recent studies on the use of laboratory findings to determine need for further imaging for intra-abdominal injury

Study	No. of patients	Type	UA	AST/ALT	CBC	COAGS
Holmes [2]	1095	Prospective	OR 4.8 Microscopic UA + for IAI	ALT >125 or AST >200 OR 17.8	Hematocrit <30, OR 2.6	Not studied
Cotton [5]	240	Retrospective	No difference in UA for IAI	AST >131 (+PE) or ALT >101 alone had 100% sensitivity	No difference in pops	Not studied
Keller [16]	240	Retrospective	Only 8% with a negative UA had IAI	Positive in 29% of patients with IAI	Only rare abnormal	No abnormalities in isolated abdominal injuries; 43% abnormal in head injuries
Isaacman [13]	285	Retrospective	Normal UA + normal PE 100% negative predictive value	Normal PE + LFT <130: 100% negative predictive value	H/H abnormal in 8%	Not studied

Abbreviations: Coags, coagulation profile; H/H, hemoglobin/hemaocrit; PE, physical exam; Pops, either population.

Finally, there is also some literature to consider regarding pancreatic enzymes predicting pancreatic or small bowel injuries. In the review by Keller and colleagues [16], only 2% of the patients had elevated amylase and none had pancreatic injuries. In a larger study conducted by Adamson and colleagues in 2003 [25], they looked at 293 patients with torso injuries with 11% IAI in which they identified 8 patients with pancreatic injuries [20]. Only 6 of 8 patients had amylase studies performed, but 5 of those 6 had abnormal amylase levels. All of the patients who underwent CT imaging had another indication for performing CT, however (most notably abdominal pain). The authors concluded that although serial enzymes may be useful, the initial set did not help to predict injury.

When considering laboratory testing, providers should resist the temptation to order a standard panel on every patient. If the physical examination is normal and the history is still concerning, based on the previously mentioned evidence, obtaining LFTs, a CBC, and UA may help clinicians determine which child should undergo further diagnostic imaging as part of trauma evaluation. Table 1 provides a concise summary of the major studies to date and their findings.

Select organ trauma

Classic teaching has been that the spleen is the most commonly injured abdominal organ after blunt trauma in children and that the liver is the second most commonly injured organ [22]. More recently, however, in a large prospective series of 1095 patients, the liver was the most commonly injured intraabdominal organ, followed by the spleen [2]. In either case, both organs are commonly injured from blunt trauma to the abdomen in children and deserve a review of their individual injury grading systems and management. This article also discusses injuries to the intestinal tract, pancreas, and kidney.

Hepatic trauma

The diagnosis and management of liver injuries in children are important because blunt liver trauma is thought to be responsible for the greatest number of fatalities in which abdominal trauma is the primary cause of death [24]. The most common mechanisms of injury reported to result in liver injury were pedestrian struck by automobile (39%), motor vehicle collision (34%), falls or discrete blows to the abdomen (13%), bicycle injuries (5%), and nonaccidental trauma (5%) [25].

Abdominal CT scanning, particularly intravenous contrast-enhanced CT, is accurate in localizing the site and extent of liver injuries and providing vital information for treatment in patients. Trauma to the liver may result in subcapsular or intrahepatic hematoma, contusion, vascular injury, or biliary disruption. Criteria for staging liver trauma based on the American Association for the Surgery of Trauma (AAST) liver injury scale include the following:

Grade 1: Subcapsular hematoma less than 1 cm in maximal thickness, capsular avulsion, superficial parenchymal laceration less than 1 cm deep, and isolated periportal blood tracking

Grade 2: Parenchymal laceration 1–3 cm deep and parenchymal/subcapsular hematomas 1–3 cm thick

Grade 3: Parenchymal laceration more than 3 cm deep and parenchymal or subcapsular hematoma more than 3 cm in diameter

Grade 4: Parenchymal/subcapsular hematoma more than 10 cm in diameter, lobar destruction, or devascularization

Grade 5: Global destruction or devascularization of the liver

Grade 6: Hepatic avulsion [21] (CT scan grade not AAST grade)

Although it is useful to review the CT and AAST criteria for staging liver trauma, it is important to note that the hemodynamic status of a child is the primary indicator of the type of initial management required for hepatic injuries [26]. Patients with massive disruption and intractable bleeding despite aggressive fluid and blood transfusion resuscitation need emergent evaluation by a surgeon and possible exploratory laparotomy if hemodynamically unstable. As long as a child with hepatic injury remains hemodynamically stable, no emergent surgical intervention is necessary. These patients require careful management of fluid volume, however, and often require transfusion of blood. Despite careful therapy and monitoring, a percentage of initially stable children with hepatic injury are at risk of sudden exsanguination and as such should be managed under surgical supervision with bed rest, repeat serial abdominal examinations, and serial hemoglobin monitoring. The success rate of nonoperative management of pediatric liver injuries ranges from 85% to 90% [25–27]. Length and level of hospitalization and return to activity recommendations are made later in this article.

Splenic trauma

The spleen is a commonly injured abdominal organ in children who sustain blunt abdominal trauma, and splenic trauma should be suspected in children with left upper quadrant tenderness to palpation, left lower rib fractures, or evidence of left lower chest/abdominal contusion. Criteria for staging splenic trauma based on the AAST splenic injury scale include the following:

Grade 1: Subcapsular hematoma of less than 10% of surface area or capsular tear of less than 1 cm in depth

Grade 2: Subcapsular hematoma of 10%–50% of surface area, intraparenchymal hematoma of less than 5 cm in diameter, or laceration of 1–3 cm in depth and not involving trabecular vessels

Grade 3: Subcapsular hematoma of more than 50% of surface area or expanding and ruptured subcapsular or parenchymal hematoma, intraparenchymal hematoma of more than 5 cm or expanding, or laceration of more than 3 cm in depth or involving trabecular vessels

Grade 4: Laceration involving segmental or hilar vessels with devascularization of more than 25% of the spleen

Grade 5: Shattered spleen or hilar vascular injury

Because many of these injuries are self-limited in children, the management of splenic trauma has evolved to a point at which stable children are managed with bed rest, frequent examinations, serial hemoglobin monitoring, and close surgical supervision. Splenic preservation is the preferred modality to decrease the risk of postsplenectomy infection. The only absolute indication for performing a splenectomy in children is massive disruption and hemodynamic instability [26]. Conservative preservation management of splenic injuries in children has shown full recovery in 90% to 98% of patients [26,28,29].

Several reports have been cited in the literature of splenic rupture in patients with Epstein-Barr virus infection. This subset of children should be considered high risk when presenting after even minor abdominal trauma. Splenic rupture occurs in 0.1% to 0.2% of patients with infectious mononucleosis. Rupture is most likely to occur during the second and third weeks of clinical symptoms, and although it can happen spontaneously, it often has a history of recent abdominal trauma. Because bradycardia is usual in infectious mononucleosis, tachycardia is an important sign indicating possible shock in these children. Unlike most other pediatric splenic injuries, rupture of the spleen after mononucleosis usually requires surgical intervention; however, recently published data have suggested that concurrent infectious mononucleosis does not preclude the successful nonoperative management of blunt splenic injury [23].

Intestinal trauma

Fortunately, because of the inherent difficulties of establishing the diagnosis, injuries to the small intestines or colon are less common than solid organ injuries in children with blunt abdominal trauma. Holmes and colleagues [2] performed a prospective analysis of 1095 children who presented to a trauma center in which only 2% had gastrointestinal injuries identified. Injuries to the intestines include perforation, intestinal hematomas, and mesenteric tears with bleeding. They often occur as a result of deceleration trauma commonly associated with lap belt injuries. Any child in whom a "seatbelt sign" of abdominal wall contusion is present should be evaluated carefully for a minimum of 24 hours for the development of evidence of peritonitis. Many patients with a gastrointestinal injury initially have normal laboratory studies and CT scans. If a CT scan of the abdomen demonstrates pneumoperitoneum or extravasation of contrast, then this diagnosis is not difficult. More often, however, the CT scan only shows subtle signs, such as bowel wall edema. A high index of suspicion must be maintained for any child with a suspicious mechanism or examination. Abdominal pain that worsens or persists and persistent emesis must be investigated with serial examinations, judicious use of repeat abdominal CT imaging, and—at the discretion of the surgeon—exploratory laparotomy.

Pancreatic trauma

Pancreatic injuries are rare compared with other solid organ injury in children; however, injuries from falls onto the handlebar of a bicycle that result in a crush force applied to the upper abdomen are mechanisms that must induce a high index of suspicion. In one retrospective review over 14 years at a pediatric trauma center, only 26 cases of pancreatic injuries were identified, but 11 of the 26 cases were from falls onto the handlebars of a bicycle [7]. The diagnosis of pancreatic injury may be challenging. Often the laboratory and CT findings of injury to the pancreas may lag behind the clinical picture, so persistent tenderness should indicate further investigation to the clinician. The overall prognosis for pancreatic trauma is good, because several series have shown that conservative nonoperative management of pancreatic injuries without ductal disruption can result in low morbidity.

Renal trauma

If one includes the posterior abdomen and retroperitoneum in the definition of blunt abdominal trauma, then the kidney is a commonly injured solid organ in pediatric blunt abdominal trauma. The most likely cause of this type of injury is a motor vehicle collision. Like hepatic and splenic injuries, most renal traumatic injuries heal without surgical intervention; however, the combination of significant flank/abdominal trauma and hematuria (even microscopic) is indication for a CT scan to assess for renal injury. (Refer to the earlier discussion for controversies concerning screening urinanalysis in this area.)

Management and disposition

Disposition often begins with the initial medical system activation for a child suspected of having an IAI. In most states there are protocols for trauma team alert activation and triage from the field. In pediatrics this is less prominent because only 15 states specifically designate adult and pediatric trauma centers [30]. If a pediatric patient with a possible IAI does present to a hospital without any specific trauma designation, the patient should be evaluated adequately, provided stabilizing treatment as needed, and managed in accordance with advanced trauma life support (ATLS) and pediatric advanced life support (PALS) principles. Persistent vital sign instability (particularly tachycardia) is a worrisome sign and should be treated aggressively [31].

Unstable children require immediate crystalloid fluid resuscitation (20 mL/kg of normal saline or Ringer's lactate solution), and in isolated blunt abdominal trauma the following should be rapidly ordered: type and cross, CBC, LFTs, and UA [32]. Continued hemodynamic instability after two fluid boluses should be treated with transfusion of 10 mL/kg of packed red blood cells, and surgical consultation should be obtained for likely emergent laparotomy. Surgical stabilization may be necessary before a possible transfer to a referral center.

For hemodynamically stable children with a concerning mechanism of injury or abdominal examination abnormality, we recommend obtaining UA, LFTs, and a CBC [33,34]. In preverbal children if all laboratory test results are normal and the children remain hemodynamically stable, then there is no consensus on whether to perform abdominal CT imaging. Regardless of mechanism, if verbal children are alert, have normal laboratory data (eg, UA, LFTs, and CBC) without concomitant injury, or lack abdominal examination abnormality, they can be discharged safely without imaging of the abdomen. In the presence of laboratory abnormalities children should undergo CT scanning to assess for IAI.

If CT scanning is not available, the provider should transfer stable children with persistent pain or vomiting, concerning examination, or laboratory findings to a facility that can perform the needed study [35]. The provider should remember that persistent tenderness on examination or persistent emesis (even with a normal abdominal CT scan) should be taken seriously and children should be admitted to a facility with a surgeon who feels comfortable managing intestinal tract injuries in children.

Length of hospitalization and return to activity

According to consensus guidelines concerning resource use, Stylianos and colleagues [36] suggested a standardized approach to isolated spleen or liver injury and made the following recommendations . For each grade level of injury, they mandated specific days in the intensive care unit, hospital stay, imaging, and discharge activity level (normal childhood level not necessarily contact sports). For either liver or spleen grades I to III they recommended no intensive care unit stays and a total hospitalization equaling 1 day plus the level of injury. A child with a grade III spleen laceration would be hospitalized for 4 days. For grade IV

Table 2
Hospital stay and activity restriction guidelines for solid organ injury

Spleen or liver injury grade	Hospital stay	Activity restriction
Grade I–III	Injury grade + 1 day	Injury grade + 2 weeks
Grade IV	1 day intensive care unit + injury grade (for hospital day)	Injury grade + 2 weeks

Data from Stylianos S and the APSA Liver/Spleen Trauma Study Group. Compliance with evidence-based guidelines in children with isolated spleen or liver injury: a prospective study. J Pediatr Surg 2002;37(3):453–6.

injuries they recommended 1 day of intensive care unit monitoring and retaining the formula for overall hospital stay. The authors recommended no re-imaging studies regardless of injury grade, and the return to a normal age-appropriate activity level was the organ laceration grade plus 2 weeks. A child with a grade III spleen injury would be on restricted activity for 5 weeks. Their prospective validation revealed increasing compliance with this protocol and, more significantly, no adverse events when following the protocol. Only 1.9% of patients needed readmission when following these guidelines. The authors did not state the reason for readmissions in their study; however, they stated that none required an operation. Table 2 summarizes these recommendations.

Summary

Blunt pediatric trauma remains a major threat to the health and well-being of children. Management of this disease entity does not only occur in major centers—nationwide many practitioners care for children who face this issue. In this article we attempted to elucidate some key principles related to the evaluation and management of these children.

References

[1] National Center for Injury Prevention and Control. Available at: cdc.gov/ncipc/osp/charts.html. Accessed July 21, 2005.
[2] Holmes JF, Sokolove PE, Brant WE, et al. Identification of children with intra-abdominal injuries after blunt trauma. Ann Emerg Med 2002;39(5):500–9.
[3] Johnson C, Riveria FP, Soderberg R, et al. Children in car crashes: analysis of data for injury and use of restraints. Pediatrics 1994;93:960–5.
[4] Howard A, McKeag AM, Rothman L, et al. Ejections of young children in motor vehicle crashes. J Trauma 2003;55:126–9.
[5] Cotton BA, Beckert BW, Monica K, et al. The utility of clinical and laboratory data for predicting intra-abdominal injury among children. J Trauma 2004;56(5):1068–75.
[6] Machi JM, Gyuro J, Losek JD, et al. Superman play and pediatric blunt abdominal trauma. J Emerg Med 1996;14(3):327–30.
[7] Arkovitz MS, Johnson N, Garcia VN, et al. Pancreatic trauma in children: mechanisms of action. J Trauma 1997;42(1):49–53.
[8] Nadler PE, Potoka DA, Shulttz BL, et al. The high morbidity associated with handlebar injuries in children. J Trauma 2005;58(6):1171–4.
[9] Wan J, Corvino TF, Greenfield SP, et al. The incidence of recreational genitourinary and abdominal injuries in the Western New York pediatric population. J Urol 2003;170(2):1525–7.
[10] Geddes R, Irish K. Boarder belly: splenic injuries resulting from ski and snowboarding accidents. Emerg Med Australas 2005;17(2):157–62.
[11] Fort DW, Bemini JC, Johnson A, et al. Splenic rupture in hemophilia. Am J Pediatr Hematol Oncol 2003;16(3):225–9.
[12] Jona JZ, Cox-Gill J. Nonsurgical therapy of splenic rupture in a hemophiliac. J Pediatr Surg 1992;27(4):523–4.
[13] Isaacman DJ, Scarfone RJ, Kost SI, et al. Utility of routine laboratory testing for detecting intra-abdominal injury in the pediatric trauma patient. Pediatrics 1993;92(5):691–5.

[14] Jerby BL, Attorri RJ, Morton Jr D. Blunt intestinal injury in children: the role of the physical examination. J Pediatr Surg 1997;32(4):580–4.

[15] Beaver BL, Colombani PM, Fal A, et al. The efficacy of computed tomography in evaluating abdominal injuries in children with major head trauma. J Pediatr Surg 1987;22(12):1117–22.

[16] Keller MS, Colm CE, Trimble JA, et al. The utility of routine trauma laboratories in pediatric trauma resuscitations. Am J Surg 2004;188:671–8.

[17] Keller MS, Fendya DG, Weber TR, et al. Glasgow Coma Scale predicts coagulopathy in pediatric trauma patients. Semin Pediatr Surg 2001;10(1):12–6.

[18] Oldham KT, Guice KS, Kaufman RA, et al. Blunt hepatic injury and elevated hepatic enzymes: a clinical correlation in children. J Pediatr Surg 1984;19:457–61.

[19] Freeman L, Prator P. Blunt abdominal trauma in prepubertal children: ED care in the era of non-operative management. Pediatric Emergency Medicine Practice 2004;1(1):1–20.

[20] Puranik SR, Hayes JS, Long J, et al. Liver enzymes as predictors of liver damage due to blunt abdominal trauma in children. South Med J 2002;95(2):203–6.

[21] Lieu TA, Fleisher GR, Mahboubi S, et al. Hematuria and clinical findings as indicators for intravenous pyelography in pediatric blunt renal trauma. Pediatrics 1988;82(2):216–22.

[22] Stalker HP, Kaufman RA, Stedje K. The significance of hematuria in children after blunt abdominal trauma. AJR Am J Roentgenol 1990;154(3):569–71.

[23] Stein JP, Kaji DM, Eastham J, et al. Blunt renal trauma in the pediatric population: indications for radiographic evaluation. Urology 1994;44(3):406–10.

[24] Taylor GA, Eichelberger MR, Potter BM. Hematuria: a marker of abdominal injury in children after blunt trauma. Ann Surg 1988;208(6):688–93.

[25] Adamson WT, Hebra A, Thomas PB, et al. Serum amylase and lipase alone are not cost-effective screening methods for pediatric pancreatic trauma. J Pediatr Surg 2003;38:354–7.

[26] Mirvis SE, Whitley NO, Gens DR. Blunt splenic trauma in adults: CT-based classification and correlation with prognosis and treatment. Radiology 1989;171(1):33–9.

[27] Wilson RH, Moorehead RJ. Management of splenic trauma. Injury 1992;23:5–9.

[28] Meguid AA, Ivascu FA, Bair HA, et al. Management of blunt splenic injury in patients with concurrent infectious mononucleosis. Am Surg 2004;70(9):801–4.

[29] Cooper A, Barlow B, DiScala C, et al. Mortality and truncal injury: the pediatric perspective. J Pediatr Surg 1994;29:33–8.

[30] Gross M, Lynch F, Canty Sr T, et al. Management of pediatric liver injuries: a 13-year experience at a pediatric trauma center. J Pediatr Surg 1999;34:811–6.

[31] Bond SJ, Eichelberger MR, Gotschall CS, et al. Nonoperative management of blunt hepatic and splenic injury in children. Ann Surg 1996;223:286–9.

[32] Patrick DA, Bensard DD, Moore EE, et al. Nonoperative management of solid organ injuries in children results in decreased blood utilization. J Pediatr Surg 1999;34:1695–9.

[33] Konstantakos AK, Baronski AL, Plaisier BR, et al. Optimizing the management of blunt splenic injury in adults and children. Surgery 1999;126:805–12.

[34] Powell M, Courcoulas A, Gaedner M, et al. Management of blunt splenic trauma: significant differences between adults and children. Surgery 1997;122:654–60.

[35] Barnett SJ. Efficacy of pediatric specific trauma centers. Pediatr Crit Care Med 2004;5(1):93–4.

[36] Stylianos S and the APSA Liver/Spleen Trauma Study Group. Compliance with evidence-based guidelines in children with isolated spleen or liver injury: a prospective study. J Pediatr Surg 2002;37(3):453–6.

ELSEVIER
SAUNDERS

Pediatr Clin N Am 53 (2006) 257–277

PEDIATRIC CLINICS
OF NORTH AMERICA

Seizures in Children

Marla J. Friedman, DO[a],*, Ghazala Q. Sharieff, MD[b]

[a]*Division of Emergency Medicine, Miami Children's Hospital, 3100 SW 62nd Avenue, Miami, FL 33155, USA*
[b]*Children's Hospital and Health Center, University of California, San Diego, 3030 Children's Way, San Diego, CA 92123, USA*

Seizures are the most common pediatric neurologic disorder, with 4% to 10% of children suffering at least one seizure in the first 16 years of life [1]. The incidence is highest in children younger than 3 years of age, with a decreasing frequency in older children [2]. Epidemiologic studies reveal that approximately 150,000 children will sustain a first-time, unprovoked seizure each year, and of those, 30,000 will develop epilepsy [1].

A seizure is defined as a transient, involuntary alteration of consciousness, behavior, motor activity, sensation, or autonomic function caused by an excessive rate and hypersynchrony of discharges from a group of cerebral neurons. A postictal period of decreased responsiveness usually follows most seizures, in which the duration of the postictal period is proportional to the duration of seizure activity. Epilepsy describes a condition of susceptibility to recurrent seizures. The classic definition of status epilepticus refers to continuous or recurrent seizure activity lasting longer than 30 minutes without recovery of consciousness.

During a seizure, cerebral blood flow, oxygen and glucose consumption, and carbon dioxide and lactic acid production all increase. Early systemic changes include tachycardia, hypertension, hyperglycemia, and hypoxemia. Brief seizures rarely produce lasting effects on the brain. Prolonged seizures, however, can lead to lactic acidosis, rhabdomyolosis, hyperkalemia, hyperthermia, and hypoglycemia, all of which may be associated with permanent neurologic damage. Airway management and termination of the seizure are the initial priorities in patients who are actively seizing.

---

* Corresponding author.
E-mail address: mjfbabydoc@bellsouth.net (M.J. Friedman).

0031-3955/06/$ – see front matter © 2006 Elsevier Inc. All rights reserved.
doi:10.1016/j.pcl.2005.09.010
pediatric.theclinics.com

Classification of seizures

Seizures are classified as generalized or partial. Generalized seizures are associated with the involvement of both cerebral hemispheres. They may be convulsive, with prominent motor activity, or nonconvulsive. Motor involvement, when present, is usually bilateral. Generalized seizures may also involve an altered level of consciousness. Types of generalized seizures include tonic-clonic (grand mal), tonic, clonic, myoclonic, atonic-akinetic (drop attacks) or absence (petit mal) [3,4]. Generalized tonic-clonic seizures are the most common type of childhood seizure. Most tonic-clonic seizures have a sudden onset, although a small percentage of children may experience a motor or sensory aura. During the initial tonic phase, the child becomes pale, with dilation of the pupils, deviation of the eyes, and sustained contraction of muscles with progressive rigidity. Bladder or bowel incontinence is common. Clonic movements, involving rhythmic jerking and flexor spasms of the extremities, then occur. Mental status is usually impaired during the seizure and for a variable time after the seizure has ceased. Myoclonic seizures are characterized by an abrupt head drop with arm flexion and may occur up to several hundred times daily. Atonic seizures are characterized by a sudden loss of both muscle tone and consciousness. Simple (typical) absence seizures are uncommon before the age of 5 years and are characterized by a sudden cessation of motor activity, a brief loss of awareness, and an accompanying blank stare. Flickering of the eyelids may be seen. The episodes last less than 30 seconds and are not associated with a postictal period. Complex (atypical) absence seizures are usually associated with myoclonic activity in the face or extremities and an altered level of consciousness [2,3].

Partial seizures may be simple, with no impairment of consciousness, or complex, with altered mental status. Both simple and complex partial seizures may progress to secondarily generalized seizures in up to 30% of children. Simple partial seizures are associated usually with abnormal motor activity developing in a fixed pattern on the hands or face. Although simple partial seizures are associated most commonly with motor abnormalities, sensory, autonomic, and psychic manifestations also may be seen. Complex partial seizures (temporal lobe seizures) are characterized by changes in perception and sensation, with associated alterations in consciousness [3]. Seizures tend to affect the eyes (a dazed look), the mouth (lip smacking and drooling), and the abdomen (nausea and vomiting) [1]. There are other specific seizure syndromes that also occur in children.

Lennox-Gastaut syndrome has an onset between 3 and 5 years of age and is characterized by intractable mixed seizures with a combination of tonic, myoclonic, atonic, and absence seizures. Most of these children also have accompanying mental retardation and severe behavioral problems. The EEG shows an irregular, slow, high-voltage spike pattern [2,3]. Although many drugs have been used to treat this condition, management is still very difficult. Valproic acid is the drug used most commonly; however, felbamate, topiramate, lamotrigine, and zonisamide have also been used as adjunctive therapies [5,6]. The ketogenic diet has also been used with some success in these children [7].

Children between 3 and 13 years of age who suffer from benign rolandic epilepsy experience nighttime seizures during sleep. This seizure disorder is genetically inherited as an autosomal dominant trait. The initial phase of the seizure involves clonic activity of the face, including grimacing and vocalizations, which often wake the child from sleep. An electroencephalogram (EEG) is important in the evaluation of this condition because a characteristic perisylvian spiking pattern can be seen. Unless these seizures are frequent, no therapy is needed because patients usually will outgrow these episodes by early adulthood. Carbamazepine has been used with success in the treatment of frequent rolandic seizures [1–3,6].

Juvenile myoclonic epilepsy of Janz is inherited as an autosomal dominant trait that manifests in early adolescence (onset 12–18 years of age). Patients experience myoclonic jerks typically on awakening but may also have tonic-clonic (80%) or absence (25%) seizures. Typical provoking factors include stress, alcohol, hormonal changes, or lack of sleep. The EEG is helpful in the diagnosis because a pattern of fast spike-and-wave discharges can be seen. Valproic acid is the drug of choice, with lamotrigine, topiramate, felbamate, and zonisamide as alternate options [1–3,6].

Children with infantile spasms (West's syndrome) present typically between 4 and 18 months of age, with males affected more commonly than females. Up to 95% of affected children are mentally retarded, and there is a 20% mortality rate. Patients experience sudden jerking contractions of the extremities, head, and trunk. The jerking is spasmodic and often occurs in clusters. Episodes rarely occur during sleep. Up to 25% of patients have tuberous sclerosis. The EEG shows the classic pattern of hypsarrhythmia (random high-voltage slow waves with multifocal spikes) [2,3]. Treatment with adrenocorticotropic hormone (ACTH) and prednisone has been used with some success [6,8]. Valproic acid, topiramate, lamotrigine, vigabatrin, and zonisamide have also shown some effectiveness [5,6,9,10].

Differential diagnosis

A seizure represents a clinical symptom of an underlying pathologic process with many possible causes (Box 1). When a child presents with a seizure, every effort should be made to determine the cause. It is imperative to differentiate between a seizure and other nonepileptic conditions that may mimic seizure activity (Box 2). A detailed description of the event from a witness is the most important factor in an accurate diagnosis. If a historical detail does not seem typical for a seizure, an alternative diagnosis should be considered.

Nonepileptic events that involve altered levels of consciousness are common in childhood. Unlike seizures, there is no postictal phase following these episodes. Breath-holding spells affect approximately 5% of children between the ages of 6 months and 5 years. A cyanotic spell begins with a period of vigorous crying followed by breath-holding, cyanosis, rigidity, limpness, and often,

Box 1. Causes of seizures

Infectious
  Brain abscess
  Encephalitis
  Febrile seizure
  Meningitis
  Neurocysticercosis
Neurologic or developmental
  Birth injury
  Congenital anomalies
  Degenerative cerebral disease
  Hypoxic-ischemic encephalopathy
  Neurocutaneous syndromes
  Ventriculoperitoneal shunt malfunction
Metabolic
  Hypercarbia
  Hypocalcemia
  Hypoglycemia
  Hypomagnesemia
  Hypoxia
  Inborn errors of metabolism
  Pyridoxine deficiency
Traumatic or vascular
  Cerebral contusion
  Cerebrovascular accident
  Child abuse
  Head trauma
  Intracranial hemorrhage
Toxicologic
  Alcohol, amphetamines, antihistamines, anticholinergics
  Cocaine, carbon monoxide
  Isoniazid
  Lead, lithium, lindane
  Oral hypoglycemics, organophosphates
  Phencyclidine, phenothiazines
  Salicylates, sympathomimetics
  Tricyclic antidepressants, theophylline, topical anesthetics
  Withdrawals (alcohol, anticonvulsants)
Idiopathic or epilepsy
Obstetric (eclampsia)
Oncologic

Box 2. Pediatric conditions often mistaken for seizures

Disorders with altered consciousness
    Apnea and syncope
    Breath-holding spells
    Cardiac dysrhythmias
    Migraine
Paroxysmal movement disorders
    Acute dystonia
    Benign myoclonus
    Pseudoseizures
    Shuddering attacks
    Spasmus mutans
    Tics
Sleep disorders
    Narcolepsy
    Night terrors
    Sleepwalking
Psychologic disorders
    Attention deficit hyperactivity disorder
    Hyperventilation
    Hysteria
    Panic attacks
Gastroesophageal reflux (Sandifer's syndrome)

---

twitching of the extremities. A pallid spell begins with an inciting painful stimulus, followed by pallor and a brief loss of consciousness. In both types of breath-holding spells, recovery to baseline is rapid and complete. Syncope is a brief, sudden loss of consciousness usually preceded by a feeling of light-headedness. On recovery, the child may be pale and diaphoretic but responsive. Patients with atypical migraines experience altered consciousness that is often associated with blurred vision, dizziness, and a loss of postural tone [2,3,11].

Paroxysmal movement disorders involve abnormal motor activity and may mimic seizures; however, altered consciousness is rare with these events. Tics are brief, repetitive movements that may be induced by stress and are usually suppressible. Shuddering attacks are whole-body tremors lasting a few seconds with a rapid return to normal activity. Acute dystonia is characterized by an involuntary sustained contraction of the neck and trunk muscles, with abnormal posture and facial grimacing. Dystonic reactions in children are seen most often as a side effect of certain medications. Pseudoseizures may present with a variety of paroxysmal movements, may be difficult to distinguish from a true seizure, and are often seen in children who have a relative with epilepsy or in patients who have a true seizure disorder. Features suggestive of a pseudoseizure include a lack of coordination of movements, moaning or talking during the episode, the absence of incontinence or bodily injury, and suggestibility. Benign myoclonus is marked by self-limited, sudden jerking movements of the extremities, usually on falling asleep. Spasmus nutans occurs in children 4 to 12 months of age and causes head tilt, nodding, and nystagmus. Infants with Sandifer's syndrome (gastroesophageal reflux) present with crying, vomiting, and writhing, arching movements of the neck and back [2,3,11,12].

Some nonepileptic paroxysmal events are associated with sleep and can be differentiated from seizures by their characteristic alterations in behavior. Night terrors occur in the preschool-aged child, with a sudden awakening from sleep, followed by crying, screaming, and inconsolability. The child then returns to sleep and has no recollection of the event. Sleepwalking (somnambulism) is seen in school-aged children who awaken from sleep with a glassy stare and walk around aimlessly for several seconds. The child then falls back asleep easily on returning to bed. Narcolepsy often presents in adolescence with an abrupt change of alertness and uncontrollable daytime sleepiness. Oftentimes, narcolepsy is associated with cataplexy, the sudden loss of muscle tone with preservation of consciousness [2,3,11].

History and physical examination

Obtaining a detailed history is critical in the evaluation of a seizure because of the many possible causes of a seizure as well as the numerous conditions that can simulate a seizure. The history should focus on both the events immediately before the onset of the episode as well as a thorough description of the actual seizure. The information to elicit includes the duration, movements, eye findings, cyanosis, loss of consciousness, the presence of an aura, incontinence, length of the postictal period, and any post-seizure focal neurologic abnormalities. Further information to obtain includes potential precipitating factors such as trauma, ingestion, recent immunizations, fever, or other systemic signs of illness. Home therapies for any recent illnesses should also be determined. If it is known that the child has a seizure disorder, then it is important to ascertain whether the recent seizure was different from previous seizures, the typical seizure frequency for the patient, any medications the patient is taking, and whether the patient has been compliant with the medication regimen or there have been any recent medication changes. Additional history to elicit includes other significant medical problems (neurologic disease, presence of a ventriculoperitoneal [VP] shunt, or developmental delay), recent travel history, and a family history of seizures.

A thorough physical and neurologic examination should be performed. Vital signs, including temperature, heart rate, and blood pressure, should be obtained. Fever is the most common cause of seizures in children (as discussed later). The head should be examined for microcephaly, dysmorphic features, signs of trauma, and the presence of a VP shunt. In infants, a measurement of the head circumference may be helpful. A bulging fontanelle indicates increased intracranial pressure. The eyes should be examined for papilledema and retinal hemorrhages. Evaluate the neck for signs of meningeal irritation. The presence of hepatospleno-megaly may indicate a metabolic or glycogen storage disease. Assess the skin for lesions such as *café au lait* spots (neurofibromatosis), adenoma sebaceum or ash leaf spots (tuberous sclerosis), and port wine stains (Sturge-Weber syndrome). Unexplained bruising should raise the suspicion of a bleeding disorder or child abuse [3].

Diagnostic approach

Laboratory testing

Laboratory testing for a child who has an afebrile seizure should be guided by the history and physical examination. A rapid bedside glucose test should be performed. A drug level should be obtained in patients who are taking anti-convulsant medications [4]. The determination of serum electrolytes, calcium, magnesium, ammonia, white blood cell count, and toxicology screens may not be necessary in a child who is alert and has returned to a baseline level of function and should be based on clinical suspicion [13]. In patients who have no iden-tifiable risk factors, an accurate and thorough history and physical examination have been shown to yield more diagnostic information than a laboratory evalua-tion [14]. However, newborns and infants less than 6 months of age have been found to be at a greater risk for electrolyte abnormalities because of underlying metabolic abnormalities, specifically hyponatremia resulting from the increased free water intake from formula overdilution [15]. Patients who have abnormal electrolyte values are more likely to have been actively seizing on presentation, have hypothermia (temperature less than 36.5°C), or be younger than 1 month of age [16]. A temperature lower than 36.5°C has been shown to be the best predictor of hyponatremia-induced seizures in infants younger than 6 months of age [17]. Based on the results of these reports, it is reasonable to obtain laboratory studies on pediatric patients who have prolonged seizures, are younger than 6 months of age, have a history of diabetes, metabolic disorder, dehydration, or excess free water intake, and patients who have an altered level of consciousness.

Routine lumbar puncture is not indicated in patients who are alert and oriented after a first afebrile seizure. A lumbar puncture should be considered after neonatal seizures occur and should be performed in patients who have an altered mental status, signs of meningeal irritation, or a prolonged postictal period [13].

Neuroimaging

Emergent neuroimaging typically is not necessary in well-appearing children after a first, unprovoked nonfebrile seizure [13]. Radiologic imaging of the seizure patient in an emergency setting usually consists of a computed CT scan of the brain. A CT scan is indicated in the acute evaluation of patients who have a focal seizure or persistent seizure activity, a focal neurologic deficit, a VP shunt, a neurocutaneous disorder, signs of elevated intracranial pressure, and a history of trauma or travel to an area endemic for cysticercosis. Patients who have immuno-compromising diseases (malignancy or HIV), hypercoagulable states (sickle cell disease), or bleeding disorders are also candidates for emergent imaging [18,19]. A MRI study is more sensitive than a cranial CT scan for the detection of certain tumors and vascular malformations. However, MRI is not readily available on an emergent basis [3,4]. Emergent imaging should be performed only in patients who have high-risk criteria. Low-risk patients can be discharged for follow-up without undergoing immediate imaging [13].

Electroencephalography

An EEG is rarely needed in the acute setting, except for patients who have refractory seizures or in patients in whom the diagnosis of nonconvulsive status epilepticus is being considered. Well-appearing children who have experienced a first-time afebrile seizure should be referred for outpatient EEG testing [3,4]. An ictal EEG taken during a seizure event is most useful, but because this is not always possible, a complete EEG recording should include both sleep and wake cycles as well as periods of patient stimulation. It is important to note, however, that a normal EEG does not rule out epilepsy or other underlying neurologic disorders [20].

Management

Acute stabilization

Status epilepticus should be considered in any patient who presents to an acute care setting with active seizure activity. An algorithm for the management of status epilepticus is presented in Fig. 1. The initial management should focus on the stabilization of the airway, breathing, and circulation and stopping the seizure. The patient should be positioned to allow for an open airway, and if necessary, an oral or nasal airway should be inserted. Oxygen should be administered and further equipment for assisted ventilation should be at the bedside. Intravenous (IV) access should be established promptly. The actively convulsing patient should also be protected from self-inflicted trauma. A rapid glucose level de-termination should be performed at the bedside, and a glucose infusion should be initiated for documented hypoglycemia. Dextrose should not be given empirically to children on ketogenic diets because this will break the ketogenic state and may result in increased seizure activity. Naloxone should be administered in cases of suspected drug exposures. The dministration of pyridoxine should be considered in neonates and those with possible isoniazid ingestion [21–24].

Most patients who present with active convulsions will require pharmacologic treatment to end the seizure. Benzodiazepines are the initial drugs of choice for

Establish ABCs: Maintain airway, give oxygen, support ventilation, establish IV access

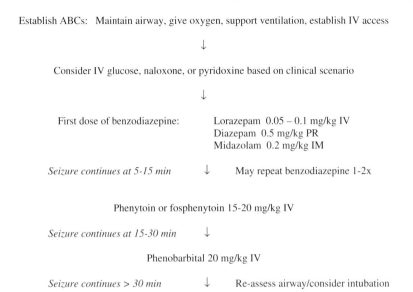

Fig. 1. An algorithm for the management of status epilepticus. ABC, airway, breathing, circulation; PR, administered rectally.

the acute management of seizures [21,24]. Lorazepam is the preferred agent because of its rapid onset (2–5 minutes) and long half-life (12–24 hours). It can be given in the IV or intramuscular (IM) form at a dose of 0.05 to 0.1 mg/kg (maximum 4 mg/dose). The dose may be repeated after 5 to 15 minutes, but the drug's effectiveness decreases with subsequent doses [4,24]. Diazepam has a rapid onset but a much shorter half-life (less than 30 minutes) than lorazepam. If diazepam is given for seizure termination, a long-term agent should be used in addition to prevent seizure recurrence. Diazepam can be given in a dose of 0.2 to 0.4 mg/kg IV or intraosseous (IO) (maximum 10 mg/dose). If IV access is not readily available, diazepam can also be given rectally, administering the IV formulation at a dose of 0.5 mg/kg [24–26]. Another agent to consider is midazolam, which can be administered by many routes, including IV, IM, rectal, intranasal, and buccal [24,26–28]. The major side effects of the benzodiazepines are respiratory depression and sedation, especially with repeated doses or in combination with a barbiturate.

Phenytoin or fosphenytoin is administered if a seizure continues despite the use of benzodiazepine. Phenytoin can only be instilled by IV at a loading dose of 10 to 20 mg/kg, with each 1 mg/kg of drug given, raising the serum concentration by 1 mg/mL. Phenytoin has a peak effect at 10 to 20 minutes after completion of the infusion and a duration of action of 12 to 24 hours. Phenytoin must be administered slowly (0.5–1.0 mg/kg/min to a maximum of 50 mg/kg/min) and under cardiac monitoring because of the risk of hypotension and cardiac dysrhythmias with rapid infusion. Furthermore, it cannot be mixed in a dextrose-

Table 1
Common anticonvulsant agents

Drug	Indication	Side effects	Maintenance (mg/kg/d)
Carbamazepine (Tegretol)	Generalized tonic-clonic, partial, benign rolandic seizures	Rash, hepatitis, diplopia, aplastic anemia, leukopenia	10-40 mg/kg/day
Clonazepam (Klonopin)	Myoclonic, akinetic, partial seizures, infantile spasms, Lennox-Gastaut	Fatigue, behavioral issues, salivation	0.05–0.30
Ethosuximide (Zarontin)	Absence	GI upset, weight gain, lethargy, SLE, rash	20–40
Felbamate (Felbatol)	Refractory severe epilepsy	Aplastic anemia, hepatotoxicity	15–45
Gabapentin (Neurontin)	Partial and secondarily generalized seizures	Fatigue, dizziness diarrhea, ataxia	20–70
Lamotrigine (Lamictal)	Complex partial, atonic, myoclonic, absence, tonic-clonic, Lennox-Gastaut, infantile spasms	Headache, nausea, rash, diplopia, Stevens-Johnson synd, GI upset	5–15
Levetiracetam (Keppra)	Adjunctive therapy for refractory partial seizures	Headache, anorexia, fatigue, infection	10–60
Oxcarbazepine (Trileptal)	Adjunctive therapy for partial seizures	Fatigue, low sodium, nausea, ataxia, rash	10–45
Phenobarbital (Luminol)	Generalized tonic-clonic, partial, myoclonic	Sedation, behavioral issues	2–6
Phenytoin (Dilantin)	Generalized tonic-clonic, partial, atonic, myoclonic, neonatal	Gum hyperplasia, hirsutism, ataxia, Stevens-Johnson syndrome, lymphoma	4–8
Primidone (Mysoline)	Generalized tonic-clonic, partial	Rash, ataxia, behavioral issues, sedation, anemia	10–25
Tiagabine (Gabitril)	Adjunctive therapy for refractory complex partial (focal) seizures	Fatigue, headache tremor, dizziness, anorexia	Titrate from 0.10 mg/kg/d; avg. dose 6 mg/d
Topiramate (Topamax)	Refractory complex partial seizures, adjunctive therapy for temporal lobe epilepsy	Fatigue, nephrolithiasis, ataxia, headache, tremor, GI upset	1–9
Valproic acid (Depakote)	Generalized tonic-clonic, absence, myoclonic, partial, akinetic, infantile spasms	GI upset, liver involvement, tremor, alopecia, sedation, weight gain	10–60
Vigabatrin (Sabril)	Infantile spasms, adjunctive therapy for refractory seizures	Weight gain, behavior changes, visual field constriction	30–150
Zonisamide (Zonegran)	Adjunctive therapy for partial seizures, atonic, infantile spasms	Fatigue, ataxia, anorexia, GI upset, headache, rash	2–8

Abbreviation: SLE, systemic lupus erythematosus.

containing solution because of precipitation problems. Local reactions such as thrombophlebitis are common following infusion, and tissue necrosis may be seen with accidental infiltration [4,21–24]. Fosphenytoin is a prodrug developed recently whose active metabolite is phenytoin. Its advantages include a more rapid administration (3 mg/kg/min to a maximum of 150 mg/min), fewer local and systemic side effects, the option of IM injection, and the ability to give the drug in a saline or dextrose-containing solution. The drug is dosed as phenytoin equivalents (PE) with a loading dose of 10 to 20 mg of PE/kg [4,24,29].

Phenobarbital is the next drug to be added if seizures persist. In neonates, however, phenobarbital is the initial drug of choice. It is given in a loading dose of 20 mg/kg, with an onset of action in 15 to 20 minutes and an anticonvulsant duration effect of between 24 and 120 hours. It causes significant sedation, hypotension, and respiratory depression, especially when used in conjunction with a benzodiazepine [4,21–24].

Continuous infusions of pentobarbital, midazolam, or propofol may be needed for refractory seizures. The patient should be ventilated mechanically and have continuous EEG monitoring. The medication should be titrated to maintain a flat-line or suppression pattern on the EEG. If seizures continue for more than 1 hour despite the above therapies, patients may require general anesthesia, neuro-muscular blockade, and continuous EEG monitoring in an intensive care setting [3,21–23].

Long-term treatment

The decision to initiate treatment with an anticonvulsant medication is based on many factors. Considerations include the patient's age, type of seizure, risk of recurrence, and other predisposing medical issues. Maintenance medications are usually not initiated for stable, well-appearing children after a single afebrile seizure. Although anticonvulsant agents may decrease the incidence of a second seizure, they do not reduce the long-term risk of developing epilepsy. Patients who experience recurrent seizures, however, should be started on an antiepileptic medication. The decision to initiate long-term anticonvulsant therapy should be made in conjunction with the patient's primary care provider or a neurologist [13,20,30].

There are numerous agents available to prevent pediatric seizures (Table 1). Several guidelines have been suggested to aid in the choice of an anticonvulsant medication [3,10,31].

1. Choose an agent that is effective for the particular type of seizure. If several drugs are available, use the drug that is least toxic.
2. Initiate therapy with a single agent.
3. Start at the low end of the dosage range.
4. Continue the same drug for at least long enough to reach a steady state, usually five times the half-life of the drug.

5. Increase the dosage until seizure control is achieved or unacceptable side effects occur.
6. Consider adding another agent if the patient continues to have seizure activity. Aim for a goal of monotherapy by eventually eliminating the first drug.

Carbamazepine (Tegretol) is useful for treating generalized tonic-clonic, simple, and complex partial seizures. It is also the drug of choice for treating benign rolandic epilepsy [2]. Recommended maintenance doses range from 10 to 40 mg/kg divided into 2 or 3 daily doses. Doses should be started at 5 mg/kg/d and increased by 5 mg/kg every 3 to 4 days until an effective maintenance level is achieved. Therapeutic serum levels range from 4 to 12 µg/mL. Dose-related adverse effects include drowsiness, blurred vision, and lethargy. Other side effects include rash, leukopenia, aplastic anemia, and hepatic toxicity. Toxic carbamazepine levels may result from the concomitant use of macrolide antibiotics, cimetidine, isoniazid, and certain calcium channel blockers. Carbamazepine may also interfere with the effectiveness of oral contraceptives [30–32].

Phenytoin (Dilantin) is effective against generalized tonic-clonic and both types of partial seizures. The usual maintenance dose ranges from 4 to 8 mg/kg/d given once, twice, or three times daily. Therapeutic serum levels range from 10 to 20 µg/mL. Because of varying rates of absorption of the drug, small dosage changes can result in large changes in serum drug levels. Similarly, drug levels may also be affected if either the trade or generic form of the drug is substituted for the other. Nondose-dependent adverse effects include gingival hyperplasia, hirsutism, and acne. These cosmetic side effects may limit the drug's long-term use, especially in girls. Other side effects include drug-induced rashes (Stevens-Johnson syndrome) and blood and liver toxicity. Dose-related toxic effects, such as nausea, vomiting, drowsiness, ataxia, and nystagmus, usually occur with levels outside the therapeutic range. Phenytoin can interfere with the effectiveness of other anticonvulsant agents, decreasing serum levels of carbamazepine, clonazepam, and primidone, and increasing the serum concentration of phenobarbital. The administration of cimetidine, estrogens, chlorpromazine, chloramphenicol, isoniazid, and anticoagulants may result in an increased phenytoin drug level [24,30–32].

Phenobarbital (Luminol) is useful for treating generalized tonic-clonic and partial seizures and is a first-line agent for treating neonatal seizures. The usual dose ranges from 2 to 6 mg/kg/d, given once or twice daily, with a therapeutic range of 10 to 40 µg/mL. Phenobarbital is fairly inexpensive and so is used commonly as a the initial drug. However, it does have several undesirable side effects in 30 to 50% of children who experience hyperactivity, mood alterations, cognitive dysfunction, and sleep problems. These common behavioral effects cause many clinicians to limit the use of this drug [24,30,32].

Primidone (Mysoline) is metabolized to phenobarbital, so the two drugs are useful for treating the same types of seizures, and both cause similar side effects. The usual dose is between 10 and 25 mg/kg/d, given in two to four divided doses.

Maintenance doses should be started at the low end of the dosage range because excessive sedation and ataxia are common at higher doses. The therapeutic range is between 5 and 12 μg/mL and is measured by monitoring the serum level of phenobarbital [30–32].

Valproate (Depakote) is quite effective for the treatment of absence and myoclonic seizures but can be used for generalized tonic-clonic and partial seizures as well. Valproic acid has also been used with success in the treatment of Lennox-Gastaut seizures, juvenile myoclonic epilepsy of Janz, and occasionally in the management of infantile spasms [2,5]. The typical maintenance dose ranges from 10 to 60 mg/kg/d, divided two to four times daily. Daily doses should be initiated at 10 mg/kg and increased by 10 mg/kg weekly until a therapeutic serum level of 50 to 100 μg/mL is established. Common side effects include gastrointestinal (GI) upset, weight gain, drowsiness, and alopecia. Tremors and thrombocytopenia are dose-related effects. Children less than 2 years of age are at an increased risk for liver and pancreatic toxicity. Valproate interferes with the metabolism of other anticonvulsant agents and may increase the drug levels of phenobarbital, phenytoin, carbamazepine, diazepam, clonazepam, and ethosuxamide [30–32].

Ethosuxamide (Zarontin) is most effective for the treatment of absence seizures. The maintenance dose ranges from 20 to 40 mg/kg/d, divided into two daily doses, with an optimal therapeutic serum level of 40 to 100 μg/mL. Common side effects include GI upset, weight gain, and headache, with the rare occurrence of erythema multiforme and a lupus-like syndrome [30,31].

Clonazepam (Klonopin) is useful for the management of myoclonic and atonic seizures. The usual dose is 0.05 to 0.3 mg/kg/d, given in two to four divided doses, with a therapeutic range of 0.02 to 0.08 μg/mL. Side effects include drowsiness, ataxia, and drooling [31,32].

Lamotrigine (Lamictal) is indicated for the management of partial, atonic, myoclonic, and tonic seizures, as well as Lennox-Gastaut syndrome. The maintenance dose ranges from 5 to 15 mg/kg/d, but because the drug interferes with other anticonvulsant agents, the dosage should be adjusted when used in conjunction with other antiepileptic medications. Lamictal should be initiated at low doses in patients who are also taking valproic acid and at higher doses when used in conjunction with phenytoin, carbamazepine, phenobarbital, or primidone. Lamictal is generally well tolerated, with most side effects being transient or dose-related, including GI upset, somnolence, dizziness, headache, and diplopia. The adverse effect of most concern is the development of a rash (Stevens-Johnson syndrome), which is especially common in patients who are also taking valproic acid [6,10,24,30,33].

Felbamate (Felbatol) is used mainly to treat intractable seizures that are refractory to other treatments, mainly the seizures of Lennox-Gastaut syndrome. The usual dose is 15 to 45 mg/kg, divided three to four times daily. It should be started at the low end of the dosage range and should be used as monotherapy because the risk of adverse effects is increased when it is used with other agents. Felbamae is known to increase the serum concentrations of phenobarbital, phenytoin, and valproic acid and to decrease that of carbamazepine. Side effects include anorexia, nausea, vomiting, insomnia, and lethargy, with the major adverse effects of aplastic anemia and severe hepatotoxicity being reported as well. Children taking this medication should have blood counts and liver enzymes monitored frequently [6,10,30,33].

Gabapentin (Neurontin) is indicated for the management of partial and secondarily tonic-clonic seizures at a dose of 20 to 70 mg/kg/d. The dose should be given three to four times daily because of the drug's short half-life. A major advantage of gabapentin is its lack of notable adverse effects. Minor side effects may include fatigue, dizziness, ataxia, and diarrhea. Increased appetite and weight gain may also occur [6,10,24,30,33].

Vigabatrin (Sabril) is effective for treating refractory partial seizures and infantile spasms. The maintenance dose is between 30 and 150 mg/kg/d, given once or twice daily. If seizures do not improve while on the drug, the patient is considered to be resistant to the drug. In some infants who have infantile spasms, treatment with vigabatrin resulted in the development of partial seizures, which is considered by some experts to be an improvement. The most impressive response has been seen in infants with tuberous sclerosis, with an efficacy similar to ACTH [10]. Side effects include weight gain, hyperactivity, and behavioral changes. The development of visual field constriction is a serious side effect that has limited the use of this drug [6,10,24,30].

Topiramate (Topamax) is indicated as adjunctive therapy in treating children with partial or generalized tonic-clonic seizures. It has also been effective in the treatment of Lennox-Gastaut syndrome, infantile spasms, and refractory complex partial seizures. The initial dose starts at 1 mg/kg/d, with a target maintenance dose of 3 to 9 mg/kg/d. The drug's interaction with other anticonvulsant agents is minor. Topiramate produces several adverse effects of concern, with behavioral problems being the most common in children. Other side effects include anorexia, weight loss, sleep problems, fatigue, headache, diplopia, speech problems, and confusion. Nephrolithiasis is another serious effect of topiramate, and its use should be carefully considered in patients who have a history of kidney stones or those on a ketogenic diet [6,10,24,30,33].

Tiagabine (Gabitril) is indicated as adjunctive therapy for managing refractory partial seizures. Dosing should begin at 0.1 mg/kg/d and be adjusted to a target dose of 0.5 to 1 mg/kg/d until adequate seizure control is achieved. Adverse effects are dose-related and more common with polytherapy. Reported side effects include fatigue, dizziness, headache, difficulty concentrating, and depressed mood [6,10,24,30,33].

Levetiracetam (Keppra) is effective as adjunctive therapy for refractory partial seizures in children aged 6 to 12 years of age. Usual maintenance doses range from 10 to 60 mg/kg/d. Adverse effects in the pediatric population include headache, anorexia, fatigue, and infection, including rhinitis, otitis media, gastroenteritis, and pharyngitis. Leukopenia has been reported in the adult literature but no such effect has been demonstrated in children [6,33].

Oxcarbazepine (Trileptal) is indicated as adjunctive therapy for treating partial seizures in children. Initial dosing begins at 5 mg/kg/d and is titrated upward, as needed, to 45 mg/kg/d. Serum concentrations of phenobarbital and phenytoin may be increased when used in conjunction with oxcarbazepine. Adverse effects include somnolence, nausea, ataxia, diplopia, and a hypersensitivity rash. Approximately 25% of children who have had an allergic reaction to carbamazepine will develop a similar reaction to oxcarbazepine [6,33].

Zonisamide (Zonegran) is indicated as adjunctive therapy against partial seizures in children 16 years of age and older. It is also effective against generalized tonic-clonic, myoclonic, and atonic seizures as well as treatment for infantile spasms and Lennox-Gastaut syndrome. The initial dose is 2 to 4 mg/kg/d, given two or three times daily, with a maintenance range of 4 to 8 mg/kg/d. Common side effects include fatigue, GI upset, anorexia, ataxia, and rash. Adverse effects are more common early in the course of therapy and are less problematic with gradual dosage adjustments [6,33].

The ketogenic diet should be considered in children with refractory tonic, myoclonic, atonic, and atypical absence seizures whose seizures have failed to respond to standard anticonvulsant therapy. This diet has also been effective in the treatment of infantile spasms and Lennox-Gastaut syndrome. Studies have demonstrated a 50% to 70% reduction in seizures in children on the ketogenic diet [6,7]. The premise of therapy is that starvation will produce a ketosis that is associated with seizure reduction. The therapy is initiated with a 5- to 7-day inpatient hospital stay during which starvation is instituted until ketosis is achieved. Hypoglycemia is common during this starvation phase, and blood glucose levels must be aggressively monitored. Vomiting and dehydration may also occur during this initiation phase. A diet of 3 to 4 parts fat to 1 part carbohydrate and protein is then introduced. Vitamin and mineral deficiencies should be avoided with appropriate supplementation. Metabolic abnormalities that may develop include renal tubular acidosis, hypoproteinemia, and elevated lipids and hepatic and pancreatic enzymes. Other effects include infection and prolonged QT intervals. Therefore, an EKG and metabolic evaluation (including evaluation for inborn errors of metabolism) should be performed before initiating the diet. Laboratory studies should be monitored routinely during therapy as well [3,6,24].

Disposition

Well-appearing children may be managed following a first-time afebrile seizure on an outpatient basis, with the appropriate follow-up. Seizure first aid should be explained to the family before discharge. These children do not require anticonvulsant therapy, but they should be scheduled for EEG testing [3]. The overall recurrence rate in children with a first unprovoked afebrile seizure varies from 14% to 65%, with most recurrences seen in the first 2 years after the initial event [10,14]. The EEG has been found to be the most important predictor of recurrence, with a 2-year recurrence rate of 58% in patients who have an abnormal EEG result compared with a 28% seizure recurrence rate in patients who have a normal EEG result [34].

The decision to initiate drug therapy and the choice of anticonvulsant agent should be made in conjunction with the patient's primary care provider and, oftentimes, in consultation with a neurologist [14]. These choices are complicated and should consider the risks associated with a seizure (recurrence, chance of injury, and psychosocial implications) against those of drug therapy (toxicity, effects on behavior and intelligence, and expense) [2,3]. Children with a prolonged seizure or postictal state or status epilepticus should be hospitalized for further observation and evaluation.

Special considerations

Neonatal seizures

It is often difficult in the newborn to differentiate between a seizure from other conditions, especially because newborns' seizures can present in a variety of different ways, including apnea, subtle eye deviations, or abnormal chewing movements. In addition, associated autonomic system findings seen commonly with older seizure patients may not be apparent in neonates. A useful tip in differentiating between a newborn who has a seizure and a "jittery baby" is that true seizures cannot be suppressed by passive restraint, whereas seizures cannot be elicited by motion or startling [35].

The most common cause of a seizure in the first 3 days of life is perinatal hypoxia or anoxia. Approximately 50% to 65% of newborn seizures are caused by hypoxic-ischemic encephalopathy [36]. Intraventricular, subdural, and subarachnoid hemorrhages account for 15% of newborn seizures, and an additional 10% are caused by inborn errors of metabolism, sepsis, metabolic disorders, and toxins [37,38]. Pyridoxine deficiency is an autosomal recessive disorder that is a rare cause of newborn seizures and usually presents in the first 1 to 2 days of life [39]. These seizures will not respond to the usual therapy for status epilepticus but do respond readily to supplemental pyridoxine at a dose of 50 to 100 mg IV.

Benign familial neonatal convulsions and benign idiopathic neonatal convulsions are two types of neonatal seizures that carry a favorable prognosis. Benign familial neonatal convulsions typically present in the first 3 days of life in infants with a strong family history of epilepsy or neonatal seizures. The cause is unknown, but these seizures resolve by 1 to 6 months of age. Benign idiopathic neonatal convulsions, also known as "fifth day fits," present on the fifth day of life and cease by day 15 of life [39].

The evaluation of neonatal seizures includes a thorough investigation for an underlying cause. Cranial imaging may consist of an ultrasonogram, a head CT, or MRI. Laboratory studies including electrolytes, glucose, calcium, magnesium, toxicology screen, urinalysis and culture, complete blood count and blood culture, and cerebrospinal fluid (CSF) studies should also be obtained. If an inborn error of metabolism is suspected, then blood should be tested for amino acids, lactate, and pyruvate and ammonia levels, and urine should be tested for organic acids.

The immediate management of active neonatal seizures includes attention to the airway, breathing, and circulation and therapy to end the seizure. Benzodiazepines are often given as the first line of treatment but have been associated with serious adverse effects such as hypotension and respiratory depression in preterm and term infants, and therefore should be used with caution [38–40]. A long-acting anticonvulsant, usually phenobarbital, and then fosphenytoin are added [36]. Phenytoin is not a preferred initial agent because it has a depressive effect on the newborn myocardium and an unpredictable rate of metabolism in neonates because of immature hepatic function [38,39]. Topiramate and zonisamide are new agents that have also shown effectiveness in the treatment of neonatal seizures [35]. Pyridoxine or lidocaine may be used if refractory seizures are present [39]. If the seizure is a result of an electrolyte abnormality such as hyponatremia, hypocalcemia, or hypomagnesemia, then these abnormalities should be identified and treated rapidly. Ampicillin and either cefotaxime or gentamicin should be initiated in any patient who is suspected of having sepsis. Acyclovir also should be administered if there is a positive maternal history of herpes or the patient has a vesicular rash, focal neurologic findings, or a CSF pleocytosis or elevated CSF protein without organisms on Gram stain. Patients should be admitted to a monitored bed for further observation and evaluation [35].

Febrile seizures

Febrile seizures are the most common type of seizure in young children, with a 2% to 5% incidence of children experiencing at least one seizure before the age of 5 years [1,41]. A febrile seizure is defined as a convulsion that occurs in association with a febrile illness in children between 6 months and 5 years of age. A simple febrile seizure is single, brief ($\leq$15 minutes), and generalized. A complex febrile seizure is much less common (approximately 20%) and is recurrent in a single illness, prolonged ($\geq$15 minutes), and focal.

The peak age for febrile convulsions is between 18 and 24 months. The exact pathophysiology is unknown, but it seems that a fever lowers the seizure threshold in susceptible children. It is unclear if the seizures are related to the rate of rise of the temperature or to the absolute peak sustained temperature [41–43]. A strong genetic predisposition exists, with a family history of febrile seizures present in 25% to 40% of children with febrile seizures [24].

Most febrile seizures are benign and self-limited, with no long-term neurologic or cognitive effects identified [41–43]. Approximately one third of children who experience a first febrile seizure will have at least one recurrence, and less than 10% of children will have more than three seizures. Most recurrences (75%) occur within 1 year of the initial episode. The younger the child is at the time of the first seizure, the greater the likelihood of recurrence, with approximately 50% of children younger than 1 year of age having a recurrence [42]. Children who have higher temperatures at the time of the seizure have a lower likelihood of recurrence. A complex first febrile seizure neither alters the risk of recurrence nor predicts that recurrent seizures, if they occur, will be complex [1].

Febrile seizures occur in otherwise healthy children with no signs of meningitis, encephalitis, or other neurologic disorders. In these cases of typical febrile seizures, an extensive laboratory evaluation has been found to have low yield and is unnecessary [41]. Viral infections have been implicated in most cases in which a cause has been determined. Specifically, roseola infantum (human herpesvirus 6) and influenza A have been associated with an increased incidence of febrile seizures [44,45]. Children who have simple febrile seizures have the same risk for serious bacterial infections as children with fever alone [43,46,47].

In children younger than 1 year of age, clinical signs of meningitis may be subtle or lacking. Previous American Academy of Pediatrics guidelines recommended that a lumbar puncture (LP) be strongly considered in all infants less than 12 months of age and considered in those between 12 to 18 months of age [41]. However, a recent article [43] now recommends LP in infants less than 18 months of age only if the following are present: (1) a history of irritability, lethargy, or poor oral intake; (2) an abnormal appearance or mental status changes; (3) abnormal physical examination findings such as a bulging fontanelle, Brudzinski's sign, or severe headache; (4) any complex seizure features; (5) slow postictal clearance of mental status; and (6) pretreatment with antibiotics. Therefore, performing routine LPs in children with simple febrile seizures may no longer be necessary. EEG and cranial imaging are not routine aspects of the evaluation of a simple febrile seizure. Further diagnostic tests (blood and urine studies) should be ordered only to investigate the source of the fever based on the child's age and extent of the fever [41,46].

The treatment of a patient who presents during a febrile seizure is the same as for other seizure types. The initial priority should focus on stabilization of the airway, breathing, and circulation, with efforts then directed at terminating the seizure. The reduction of body temperature with antipyretics or other cooling methods should also be a part of the primary management. If the seizure persists, benzodiazepines are the first drug of choice. Phenytoin and phenobarbital may be used as second-line agents for persistent seizure activity [42].

Most febrile seizures, however, are brief, and patients will usually present for evaluation after the seizure activity has ceased spontaneously. For these patients, the issue of prophylactic medication therapy is controversial. The current consensus is that long-term medication therapy is not necessary for most patients who have simple febrile seizures. Following a febrile seizure, children with no other risk factors for epilepsy (a family history of epilepsy, a complex febrile seizure, or an underlying neurologic disorder) have only a 1% to 2% lifetime risk of developing epilepsy compared with a 0.5% to 1% risk in the general population [42]. In the presence of two or more of these risk factors, the future risk of developing epilepsy is 10%.

Prophylactic antipyretic therapy is not effective in reducing the risk of seizure recurrence. Anticonvulsant therapy may reduce recurrences but does not prevent the development of epilepsy. Most children with febrile seizures do not require anticonvulsant therapy. Phenobarbital has been used in the past for the long-term management of febrile seizures. To be effective, phenobarbital must be given continuously, not intermittently or at the onset of fever. Concerns about adverse behavioral and cognitive effects have limited its use. Valproic acid seems to be at least as effective as phenobarbital in preventing recurrent febrile seizures, but its association with severe hepatotoxicity in children less than 3 years of age has limited its use. Other agents, such as carbamazepine and phenytoin, are not effective in the prevention of recurrences. Oral or rectal diazepam, 0.5 mg/kg/d, given intermittently from the onset of fever has been shown to be as effective as continuous phenobarbital in preventing seizures [42]. Again, adverse effects (ataxia, lethargy, and irritability) may restrict the use of this therapy. Long-term prophylactic therapy may be considered in certain individualized cases.

Patients with a simple febrile seizure may be safely discharged to home with parental reassurance and seizure education. Those patients who have had a complex or prolonged seizure or required medication to terminate the seizure should be hospitalized.

References

[1] McAbee GN, Wark JE. A practical approach to uncomplicated seizures in children. Am Fam Physician 2000;62(5):1109–16.

[2] Vining EP. Pediatric seizures. Emerg Med Clin North Am 1994;12(4):973–88.

[3] Shneker BF, Fountain NB. Epilepsy. Dis Mon 2003;49:426–78.

[4] Reuter D, Brownstein D. Common emergent pediatric neurologic problems. Emerg Med Clin North Am 2002;20(1):155–76.

[5] Trevathan E. Infantile spasms and Lennox-Gastaut syndrome. J Child Neurol 2002;17(Suppl 2): 2S9–22.

[6] Jarrar RG, Buchhalter JR. Therapeutics in pediatric epilepsy, part 1: the new antiepileptic drugs and the ketogenic diet. Mayo Clin Proc 2003;78:359–70.

[7] Vining EP, Freeman JM, Ballaban-Gil K, et al. A multi-center study of the efficacy of the ketogenic diet. Arch Neurol 1998;55(11):1433–7.

[8] Cossette P, Riviello J, Carmant L. ACTH versus vigabatrin therapy in infantile spasms: a retrospective study. Neurology 1999;52(8):1691–4.

[9] Elterman RD, Shields WD, Mansfield KA, et al. Randomized trial of vigabatrin in patients with infantile spasms. Neurology 2001;57(8):1416–21.

[10] Marks WJ, Garcia PA. Management of seizures and epilepsy. Am Fam Physician 1998;57(7): 1589–600.

[11] Barron T. The child with spells. Pediatr Clin North Am 1991;38(3):711–24.

[12] Selbst SM, Clancy R. Pseudoseizures in the pediatric emergency department. Pediatr Emerg Care 1996;12(3):185–8.

[13] Hirtz D, Ashwal S, Berg A, Bettis D, et al. Practice parameter: evaluating a first nonfebrile seizure in children. Neurology 2000;55:616–23.

[14] Hirtz D, Berg A, Bettis D, et al. Practice parameter: treatment of the child with a first unprovoked seizure. Neurology 2003;60:166–75.

[15] Bui T, Delgado C, Simon H. Infant seizures not so infantile: first-time seizures in children under six months of age presenting to the ED. Am J Emerg Med 2002;20:518–20.

[16] Scarfone RJ, Pond K, Thompson K, et al. Utility of laboratory testing for infants with seizures. Pediatr Emerg Care 2000;16:309–12.

[17] Farrar HC, Chande VT, Fitzpatrick DF, et al. Hyponatremia as the cause of seizures in infants: a retrospective analysis of incidence, severity, and clinical predictors. Ann Emerg Med 1995; 26:42–8.

[18] Warden C, Browenstein D, Del Beccaro M. Predictors of abnormal findings of computed tomography of the head in pediatric patients presenting with seizures. Ann Emerg Med 1997; 29:518–23.

[19] Sharma S, Riviello JJ, Harper MB, et al. The role of emergent neuroimaging in children with new-onset afebrile seizures. An Pediatr (Barc) 2003;111:1–6.

[20] Scheuer ML, Pedley TA. The evaluation and treatment of seizures. N Engl J Med 1990;323: 1468–74.

[21] Lowenstein DH, Alldredge BK. Status epilepticus. N Engl J Med 1998;338:970–6.

[22] Haafiz A, Kissoon N. Status epilepticus: current concepts. Pediatr Emerg Care 1999;15:119–29.

[23] Hanhan UA, Fiallos MR, Orlowski JP. Status epilepticus. Pediatr Clin North Am 2001;48: 683–94.

[24] Wolf SM, Ochoa JG, Conway EE. Seizure management in pediatric patients for the nineties. Pediatr Ann 1998;27:653–64.

[25] Fitzgerald BJ, Okos AJ, Miller JW. Treatment of out of hospital status epilepticus with diazepam rectal gel. Seizure 2003;12:52–5.

[26] Scott RC, Besag FM, Neville BG. Buccal midazolam and rectal diazepam for treatment of prolonged seizures in childhood and adolescence: a randomized trial. Lancet 1999;353:623–6.

[27] Chamberlain JM, Altiere MA, Futterman C, et al. A prospective, randomized study comparing intramuscular midazolam with intravenous diazepam for the treatment of seizures in children. Pediatr Emerg Care 1997;13:92–4.

[28] Vilke GM, Sharieff GQ, Marino A, et al. Midazolam for the treatment of out of hospital pediatric seizures. Prehosp Emerg Care 2002;6:215–7.

[29] Wheless J. Treatment of acute seizures and status epilepticus in children. J Child Neurol 1999; 20:S47–51.

[30] Russell RJ, Parks B. Anticonvulsant medications. Pediatr Ann 1999;28:238–45.

[31] Vining EP, Freeman JM. Where, why, and what type of therapy. Pediatr Ann 1985;14:741–5.

[32] Abramowicz M. Drugs for epilepsy. Med Lett Drugs Ther 1995;37:37–40.

[33] Bergin AM. Pharmacotherapy of pediatric epilepsy. Expert Opin Pharmacother 2003;4:421–31.

[34] Shinnar S, Berg AT, Moshe SL, et al. The risk of seizure recurrence after a first unprovoked afebrile seizure in childhood: an extended follow-up. Pediatr 1996;98:216–25.

[35] Zupance ML. Neonatal seizures. Pediatr Clin North Am 2004;51:961–78.

[36] Stafstrom C. Neonatal seizures. Pediatr Rev 1995;16:248–55.

[37] Bernes S, Kaplan AM. Evolution of neonatal seizures. Pediatr Clin North Am 1994;41: 1069–104.

[38] Rennie JM, Boylan GB. Neonatal seizures and their treatment. Curr Opin Neurol 2003;16: 177–81.

[39] Evans D, Levene M. Neonatal seizures. Arch Dis Child Fetal Neonatal Ed 1998;78:F70–5.

[40] Ng E, Klinger G, Shah V, Taddio A. Safety of benzodiazepines in newborns. Ann Pharmacother 2002;36:1150–5.

[41] Provisional Committee on Quality Improvement, Subcommittee on Febrile Seizures. Practice parameter: the neurodiagnostic evaluation of the child with a first simple febrile seizure. An Pediatr (Barc) 1996;97:769–72.

[42] Committee on Quality Improvement, Subcommittee on Febrile Seizures. Practice parameter: long-term treatment of the child with simple febrile seizures. An Pediatr (Barc) 1999;103: 1307–9.

[43] Warden CR, Zibulewsky J, Mace S, et al. Evaluation and management of febrile seizures in the out of hospital and emergency department settings. Ann Emerg Med 2003;41:215–22.

[44] Chiu SS, Tse CYC, Lau YL, et al. Influenza A infection is an important cause of febrile seizures. Pediatr 2001;108:e63.

[45] Barone SR, Kaplan MH, Krilov LR. Human herpesvirus-6 infection in children with first febrile seizures. J Pediatr 1995;127:95–7.

[46] Chamberlain JM, Gorman RL. Occult bacteremia inc children with simple febrile seizures. Am J Dis Child 1988;142:1073–6.

[47] Trainor JL, Hampers LC, Krug SE, et al. Children with first-time simple febrile seizures are at low risk of serious bacterial illness. Acad Emerg Med 2001;8:781–7.

ELSEVIER
SAUNDERS

Pediatr Clin N Am 53 (2006) 279–292

Pediatric Procedural Sedation and Analgesia

Lisa Doyle, MD[a],*, James E. Colletti, MD[b]

[a]Department of Emergency Medicine, University of Arizona University Physicians Hospital,
2800 East Ajo Way, Tucson AZ 85713, USA
[b]Department of Emergency Medicine, Regions Hospital 640 Jackson Street, Mail Stop 11102F,
St. Paul, MN 55101-2502, USA

Children often present to physicians and other medical practitioners with painful conditions that require painful interventions. Procedural sedation and analgesia (PSA) refers to the pharmacologic technique of managing a child's pain and anxiety. Procedural sedation is a safe, effective, and humane way to facilitate appropriate medical care. It is important to distinguish the goal for the procedural sedation; pain relief, anxiolysis, or both. Different medications and combinations of medications can be used to achieve the desired effect. It is also important to keep in mind the possible adverse reactions and side effects associated with each medication when choosing the sedation cocktail.

The general approach to procedural sedation includes defining the goal for sedation, and assigning a qualified person to administer the appropriate sedation to an appropriate patient. One must also consider the fasting recommendations and monitoring guidelines before performing the sedation.

Definitions

Procedural sedation, as defined by the American Society of Anesthesiologists, occurs on a continuum, ranging from minimal sedation or anxiolysis to general anesthesia (Table 1). *Anxiolysis* refers to a drug-induced state in which cognitive and motor functions may be impaired. *Moderate sedation and analgesia*, also known as conscious sedation, is a state of moderate sedation in which a child

* Corresponding author.
E-mail address: lisasdoyle@gmail.com (L. Doyle).

Table 1
Sedation continuum

Status	Anxiolysis/ minimal sedation	Conscious sedation/ moderate sedation and analgesia	Deep sedation/ analgesia	General anesthesia
Responsiveness	Normal to verbal stimulation	Purposeful to verbal or light tactile stimulation	Purposeful to repeated or painful stimulation	No response to painful stimulation
Airway	Maintained	Maintained	May need intervention	Often needs intervention
Ventilation	Normal	Adequate	May need assistance	Often needs assistance
Cardiovascular function	Normal	Maintained	Usually maintained	May be impaired

responds purposefully to verbal commands with or without light tactile stimulation. Ventilatory and cardiovascular functions are unaffected during anxiolysis and moderate sedation and analgesia. *Deep sedation and analgesia* is a drug-induced depressed level of consciousness in which children respond purposefully only to repeated or painful stimulation. *General anesthesia* refers to the drug-induced loss of consciousness in which there is no response to painful stimulus. Ventilation is affected in both deep sedation and general anesthesia.

Sedation by the nonanesthesiologist

Several groups have published recommendations and guidelines directed toward the nonanesthesiologist who may perform procedural sedation [1–3]. Specific pediatric guidelines are published by the American Academy of Pediatrics (AAP) [4,5]. The most important recommendation common to all guidelines relates to the person performing the sedation. This person must be qualified to manage all potential complications, including hemodynamic instability, respiratory depression, and airway compromise. Because it is difficult to predict how an individual child will respond to a specific medication, the practitioner must be able to rescue a patient from one level greater than the intended level of sedation. For example, the practitioner performing moderate sedation for a laceration repair procedure must be able to perform airway intervention and provide ventilatory support.

Physicians routinely provide sedation and analgesia to critically ill children in the pediatric emergency department. Pitetti and colleagues [6] conducted a prospective descriptive investigation of 1215 patients and concluded that PSA can be safely and effectively provided by nonanesthesiologists. Potential arenas for the sedation of children include the pediatric emergency department, intensive care unit, subspecialty procedure suites, ambulatory surgery centers, dental offices, and physician offices. The AAP Committee on Drugs guidelines applies to all settings of pediatric procedural sedation. All sites should have age- and size-appropriate equipment and medications immediately available. Sites other than hospitals should have a protocol for access to back-up emergency services, and ready access to ambulance service must be assured [4,5].

Equipment and monitoring

The practice guidelines and clinical policies cited above describe the supportive equipment and monitors that must be available when performing pediatric procedural sedation. Equipment must be age- and size-appropriate and include oxygen, suction, medications, a bag-mask ventilation device, and intubation equipment. Necessary monitors include pulse oximetry and cardiac monitors with appropriate alarms. Blood pressure should be determined before sedation begins and at 5-minute intervals during sedation. An exception to this guideline is when the blood pressure measurement interferes with the sedation, as in the case of giving minimal sedation to a child undergoing radiologic procedures.

Respiratory depression is the most serious unwanted side effect of most medications used in procedural sedation. The detection and recognition of respiratory depression is one of the most important aspects of monitoring. The use of supplemental oxygen can decrease the usefulness of pulse oximetry as a measure for hypoventilation. Instead, the observation of chest rise or ausculta-tion of lung sounds is necessary to detect respiratory depression. To overcome this difficulty in cases in which access to a patient's chest wall is suboptimal, capnography was developed. The measurement of exhaled carbon dioxide is a noninvasive monitoring technique developed for use by anesthesiologists in the operating room. Respiratory gases are sampled in-line from an endotracheal tube or side-stream at the nares. A waveform is produced by variations in the level of carbon dioxide during the respiratory cycle. End-tidal carbon dioxide is highest during expiration and lowest during inspiration. The relationship between the exhaled carbon dioxide and the arterial partial pressure of carbon dioxide is linear. Changes in a child's measured carbon dioxide level or loss of the wave-form indicates hypoventilation or apnea.

The measurement of exhaled carbon dioxide has been applied successfully in outpatient oral surgery, endoscopy, intensive care unit, MRI, and emergency department settings [7–12]. Studies have shown that capnography, the continuous measurement and display of carbon dioxide, is reliable in predicting respiratory depression. The measurement of end-tidal carbon dioxide should be considered for all children receiving deep sedation and for patients whose ventilation cannot be observed directly during moderate sedation.

Miner and colleagues [13] recently studied the use of end-tidal carbon dioxide monitoring as a means to predict the level of sedation in emergency department patients undergoing procedural sedation. Although the investigators did validate the use of capnography in detecting respiratory depression, they did not find that end-tidal carbon dioxide predicts the level of sedation. To deal with this aspect of monitoring, another technology, bispectral index monitoring, is making the transition from operating room to the outpatient setting.

Table 2
Medications for sedation and analgesia

Drug (class)	Indications	Absolute contraindications (in addition to hypersensitivity)	Relative contraindications	Unpleasant effects
Morphine (opioid)	Analgesia; may cause sedation at higher dosages	—	—	Respiratory depression; hypotension; nausea; pruritus
Fentanyl (opioid)	Analgesia; may cause sedation at higher dosage	—	—	Respiratory depression; hypotension; nausea; pruritus (especially nasal)
Meperidine (opioid)	Analgesia	May cause serotonin syndrome in patients taking SSRI and MAOI	—	Active metabolite lowers seizure threshold; hypotension; long half-life
Midazolam (benzodiazepine)	Anxiolysis, sedation, antegrade amnesia	Hypotension or potential for cardiovascular collapse; narrow angle glaucoma	Renal failure, CHF	Respiratory depression; hypotension, disinhibition with paradoxical excitement
Methohexital (barbiturate)	Sedation	—	≤ 3 years old	Hypotension; respiratory depression
Pentobarbital (barbiturate)	Sedation	Liver failure; hyperactivity	Children ≥ 8 years old	Irritability; hyperactivity; nausea
Propofol (alkyl phenol)	Sedation	Egg or soy allergy; hypotension or potential for cardiovascular collapse; ≤ 3 years of age	—	Pain at injection site; hypo/hypertension; apnea

Drug				Comments
Ketamine (dissociative agent)	Dissociative state	Age ≤3 months; psychosis [35]	Elevated ICP or IOP; age ≤12 months; laryngeal stimulation; laryngospasm; URI; active asthma; cardiac disease; porphyria; thyroid disease; seizure disorder [21]	Unpleasant emergent reaction; random movements may occur, therefore not ideal for CT or MRI sedation; hypersalivation; laryngospasm; nausea
Etomidate (hypnotic imidazole derivative)	Sedation with tenuous hemodynamic status	Seizure disorder; age ≤12 years old	Other sedation strategies may be more appropriate in children	Myoclonus; pain at injection site
Diphenhydramine (antihistamine)	Sedation, adjunct to opioids to prevent histamine release	Nonreversible; do not use if a child's neurologic status needs to be followed; neonates; premature infants	—	May cause hallucination in overdose
Chloral hydrate (sedative hypnotic)	Sedation	Nonreversible; do not use if a child's neurologic status needs to be followed	Age ≥3 years	Erratic mucosal absorbtion; paradoxical excitement; may predispose to airway obstruction
Nalaxone (opioid antagonist)	Reverse opioids	—	—	—
Flumazenil (benzodiazepine antagonist)	Reverse benzodiazepines	Benzodiazepine use ≥2 wk; increased ICP	—	—

Abbreviations: CHF, congestive heart failure; ICP, intracranial pressure; IOP, intraocular pressure; MAOI, monoamineoxidase inhibitor; SSRI, selective serotonin reuptake inhibitor; URI, upper respiratory infection.

Bispectral index monitoring is a noninvasive electronic method of evaluating a patient's level of sedation. The bispectral index score (BIS) uses electroencephalogram signals that are recorded on a self-adhesive forehead probe. Electroencephalographic waveforms change with a child's level of alertness. The BIS is a numerical score of 1 to 100, with 1 being no brain activity and 100 being fully awake. This has been used in pediatric oral surgery, endoscopy, and adult emergency department settings to monitor sedation [14–16]. Optimal BIS scores are reported between 45 for pediatric patients to as high as 85 in adults [17,18]. An important application of the BIS technology appears to be in alerting the clinician when a patient reaches a deep level of sedation. Miner and colleagues [19] found a lower rate of respiratory depression during procedural sedation when emergency physicians had access to BIS. For more information on these novel monitoring techniques, Levine and Platt [20] review the use of exhaled carbon dioxide and BIS in procedural sedation.

Sedation for a painful procedure

There are many options available to the practitioner who needs to perform sedation and analgesia for a painful procedure on a child. One option is to use a combination of intravenous medications to create a sedative and analgesic cocktail. It is important to remember the class effects of the drugs. Opioids provide pain relief but may only provide adequate sedation when used at high dosages. Using higher dosages obviously increases the risk of unwanted side effects such as respiratory depression and cardiovascular collapse. Benzodiazepines provide sedation and anxiolysis but do not provide analgesia. Propofol is also an excellent sedative but does not provide any pain relief. These classes of medication require titration to the point of general anesthesia to provide adequate analgesia for most painful procedures. Therefore, a good approach is to use opioid analgesics in combination with a sedative, an approach that is safe and effective in children [21–26].

Pena and Kraus [27] report no increase in respiratory depression with fentanyl and midazolam compared with other agents. Graff and colleagues [28] report a low incidence of respiratory events in 334 children undergoing sedation with fentanyl and midazolam. Only 11% of the children had minor respiratory events, and no patients required ventilatory assistance. In general, 10% to 20% of children have mild respiratory events under sedation and analgesia with this combination. The need for respiratory assistance is rare, and the incidence of life-threatening events in an appropriately monitored child is near zero [29].

When using a combination of medications, it is important to realize the synergistic effect the medications have with each other. The safe approach is to use a combination of only two medications. Adverse events have been related to the use of a combination of three or more mediations [30].

Ketamine is an alternative to the multidrug cocktail. Since 1990, this drug has gained popularity for pediatric emergency department sedation because it permits performing extremely painful procedures without the risk of dose-dependent cardiorespiratory depression. Ketamine dissociates the central nervous system from outside stimuli, thus producing a profound trancelike cataleptic state. The dissociative state is characterized by potent analgesia, sedation, and amnesia. This dissociation is either present or absent, and the titration of ketamine is needed only to prolong the sedation and analgesia over time. Ketamine has been proven to be a safe medication for use in children [31]. Tables 2 and 3 provide information regarding drug indications, contraindications, adverse effects, time to onset, duration of action, and dosages.

There are also many adjunct methods for providing analgesia in the pediatric population. The use of the following methods may decrease the necessary dosage of opioid analgesia, or alleviate the need altogether. Hematoma blocks provide good pain relief for distal radius fracture reduction. A eutectic mixture of local anesthetic cream or viscous lidocaine applied to the lumbar area for spinal tap anesthetizes the area well. Digital and regional nerve blocks with mild sedation are additional safe alternatives to deeper sedation and analgesia for children who present with fractures, dislocations, nail bed injuries, and lac-

Table 3
Drugs, routes, onset, and duration

Drug	Route	Time of onset (min)	Duration (min)
Morphine	IV	20 – 60	3 – 5 h
	IM	20 – 60	3 – 5 h
Fentanyl	IV	1 – 3	20 – 30
Meperidine	IV	15 – 30	3 – 4 h
Midazolam	IV	1 – 3	20 – 30
	IM	10 – 20	60 – 120
	IN	10 – 15	60
	PO	10 – 30	60 – 90
	PR	5 – 10	30 – 60
Methohexital	IV	1	10
	PR	2 – 5	45
Pentobarbital	IV	3 – 5	15 – 45
	IM	10 – 15	60 – 120
	PO and PR	15 – 60	60 – 240
Propofol	IV	1 – 2	5 – 10
Ketamine	IM	5	20 – 30
	IV	1	5 – 10
Etomidate	IV	2 – 3	20
Diphenhydramine	IV	5	2 – 6
	PO	60	4 – 6 h
Chloral Hydrate	PO and PR	15 – 30	60 – 120
Nalaxone	IV	1	15 – 30
	IM	10 – 15	60 – 90
Flumazenil	IV	1	20 – 60

Abbreviations: IM, intramuscular; IN, intranasal; PO, orally; PR, rectally; PRN, as needed.

erations. Distraction techniques used by child life specialists are also excellent adjuncts or alternatives to chemical sedation and analgesia.

Sedation for nonpainful procedures

Adequate sedation allows children to tolerate unpleasant procedures and may expedite conducting procedures that require the uncooperative child not to move. A common arena for minimal sedation is the radiology suite. Cooperation for a diagnostic study such as MRI is a frequent indication for pediatric procedural sedation. MRI scans can cause anxiety in even the most cooperative child or adult. These scans require the patient to lie still in a closed cylinder for 30 to 90 minutes, which promotes claustrophobia, while the machines make clicking and banging noises that may be particularly frightening to a child.

Medication options for nonpainful radiologic procedures include anxiolytics such as benzodiazepines and sedatives such as diphenhydramine or chloral hydrate. The practitioner must keep in mind the possible need to titrate the medication for a longer procedure such as an MRI and the need for intravenous IV access. Also, the necessity for following a child's neurologic status should be considered before administering a nonreversible sedative such as an antihistamine, chloral hydrate, or barbiturate.

Sacchetti and colleagues [32] recently published an interesting observational study regarding the need for sedation in children undergoing CT scans. They found that procedural sedation is used infrequently in infants and children undergoing fast helical CT scans of the head, face, abdomen, pelvis, and other body parts. The mean age of patients who required sedation was 23.4 months, with a median of 14 months.

Safe sedation

The Joint Commission on Accreditation of Health care Organizations (JCAHO) mandates that the standard of care for sedated children be uniform throughout an institution [33]. Although delegating the care of sedated children to a pediatric anesthesiologist may be optimal, it is not practical or cost effective.

Table 4
American Society of Anesthesiologists physical status classification

Class	Description	Suitability for sedation
1	Normal healthy patient	Excellent
2	Mild systemic disease; well-controlled chronic condition	Generally good
3	Severe systemic disease; poorly controlled chronic condition; acute illness such as pneumonia	Intermediate
4	Severe systemic disease that is a constant threat to life	Poor
5	Moribund patient who is not expected to survive without the operation	Extremely poor

Sedation by nonanesthesiologists is safe and acceptable as long as the standards of care are met, including identifying appropriate candidates for safe PSA to decrease the incidence of adverse events.

The American Society of Anesthesiologists (ASA) maintains a graded physical status classification as a useful tool for assessing a patient's appropriateness for elective procedural sedation (see Table 4). Malviya and colleagues [34] reported in 1997 that an ASA physical status of 3 or 4 and a patient who is 1 year old or less are predictors of an increased risk of sedation-related adverse events. Respiratory depression, inadequate sedation, over-sedation, and failed procedures are considered adverse events, and of these events, the most concern is for respiratory depression.

Cote and colleagues [30] published an analysis of 118 sedation-related disasters. Death and permanent neurologic injury were more likely to occur in nonhospital-based settings, despite the fact that most of these children were older and healthy. Nearly 80% of the adverse events presented initially with respiratory difficulty, and most of the unacceptable outcomes were the result of inadequate rescue and resuscitation. Adverse sedation events were associated with drug overdoses and drug interactions, particularly when three or more medications were used. Adverse events were also associated with sedative medications administered by parents at home, before medical supervision. This study underscores the importance of diligent monitoring and the necessity of a practitioner trained to intervene with cardiorespiratory depression. Box 1 lists sedation pitfalls to avoid [35].

Box 1. Procedural sedation pitfalls

Choosing a sedative when an analgesic is required
Choosing an analgesic when a sedative is required
Combining two sedative or two analgesics agents
Employing a reversal agent to speed recovery
Failure to check that the concentration of the sedative is the desired concentration
Failure to consider and discuss risk and benefits of PSA
Failure to inform family of potential adverse effects
Failure to obtain and document informed consent
Failure to properly document
Failure to write out clearly the dose and route of administration
Not having appropriate monitoring and resuscitation equipment
Not involving the services of child life specialists
Not knowing when to refer the patient to general anesthesia in the operating room
Under-sedation or over-sedation
Using a long-acting sedative agent for a brief procedure

Fasting guidelines

The practice of prolonged fasting (NPO) from solids and liquids originates from the work of Mendelson in 1946 [36]. In Mendelson's investigation, aspiration occurred in 66 of 44,016 nonfasted obstetric patients over a 13-year period. He described the risk of gastric acid aspiration during obstetric anesthesia with the consequent development of pneumonitis. Since Mendelson's article, NPO recommendations have been extrapolated to all patients requiring general anesthesia and even parenteral sedation [37]. Therefore, NPO guidelines were established by the ASA in attempt to reduce the risk of pulmonary aspiration of gastric contents.

The ASA [38] guidelines for the length of NPO before anesthesia are 6 hours after the patient receives infant formula or a light meal, 4 hours after breast milk, and 2 hours after clear liquids. These guidelines are consensus opinion-based rather than evidence-based [39]. Furthermore, the guidelines acknowledge that "there is insufficient" published evidence to address the safety of a preoperative fasting period and do not offer specific guidance for fasting times for emergency procedures [38,40].

Even though the current guidelines are consensus-based and not designed specifically for an emergency setting, a recent editorial has cautioned against disregarding or trivializing "fasting assessment before PSA. The evaluation and documentation of last oral intake is both sound medical practice and a ...JCAHO requirement" [39].

A significant challenge in the pediatric emergency department is that children are rarely fasted before presentation and often require urgent or emergent procedures. Two large prospective investigations [40,41] were undertaken to evaluate the safety of PSA without a traditional fasting period. Agrawal and colleagues [40] prospectively studied a case series of 1014 children (age 5 days to 31 years, with a median age of 5.4 years) who were undergoing PSA [41]. Data on fasting were available in 905 of the 1104 children, of whom 509 did not meet fasting guidelines. Adverse events (all minor, without an episode of aspiration) occurred in 32 (8.1%) of the 396 patients who met fasting guidelines and 35 (6.9%) of the 509 patients who did not met fasting guidelines.

Roback and colleagues [41] performed a prospective investigation of 2085 children (age 19 days to 32.1 years, with a median age of 6.7 years) who received IV PSA in a pediatric emergency department [41]. Fasting time was documented in 1555 of the 2085 patients. When the incidence of adverse events was compared among children based on fasting time in hours (0–2 hours, 2–4 hours, 4–6 hours, 6–8 hours, and ≥ 8 hours), a significant difference was not determined. Furthermore, there were no cases of aspiration discovered. Both of these studies concluded that there is no association between preprocedural fasting and the incidence of adverse events during procedural sedation.

Is a prolonged fast before PSA the best practice? Consider the following: First, the stomach of a fasting patient can produce as much as 50 mL of gastric secretions per hour [42]. Second, ingested clear liquids leave the stomach of a healthy individual rapidly, with half of the volume disappearing in 10 to 20 minutes [42]. Third, prolonged fluid deprivation has been shown to increase the volume and decrease the pH level of gastric secretions, both of which increases the likelihood and consequences of gastric acid aspiration [43,44]. Finally, a prolonged fast does not appear to decrease the incidence of emesis. Treston and colleagues [45] performed a prospective investigation of 257 children between the ages of 1 and 12 years who presented with conditions that required ED PSA with IV ketamine. Postprocedural vomiting occurred in 15.7% of 127 children who had fasted for greater than 3 hours, 14% occurred in the 100 children who had fasted for 2 to 3 hours, and 6.6% occurred in the 30 children who had fasted for 1 hour. This investigation suggested a trend toward increased vomiting with a longer fasting time. Notably, the Canadian Anaesthetists' Society has issued guidelines indicating that a fluid fast of greater than 3 hours is unnecessary in healthy patients undergoing surgery [46].

Although strict adherence to ASA procedural guidelines may not always be feasible, the practitioner should proceed with caution when not adhering to the guidelines. Significant thought should be given to the risk-benefit ratio of sedation for each patient. The presedation assessment should be balanced with the urgency of the required procedure and the anticipated depth of sedation. In cases in which the risks of proceeding are greater than the benefits, the choice of either delaying the procedure or referring the patient to the operating room for general anesthesia should be considered. In cases in which the physician decides to proceed, the safety systems already in place should be maintained and a depth of sedation in which the protective airway reflexes are impaired should be avoided, unless the benefits of such a level of sedation outweigh the risks [47].

Discharge criteria

After procedural sedation, children should not be discharged from the medical facility until they have awakened to their baseline mental and ambulatory status. Discharge instructions should be reviewed with parents or other responsible adults before the sedation and before discharge. An emphasis should be placed on the importance of watching carefully for signs of respiratory distress. Children should not be left unattended in a car seat, and a sleeping child should not be left alone. They should not participate in activities requiring coordination for 24 hours and should not swim or bathe unattended for 8 hours [48].

Summary

Procedural sedation and analgesia is a safe and effective means to manage a child's pain and anxiety. When the practitioner is deciding which methods of PSA to use, it is important to determine whether the intended goal is sedation or analgesia or both and to consider the adverse reactions and side effects of each agent. Appropriate safety measures should be undertaken, including supportive equipment, monitors, and a presedation assessment. End-tidal carbon dioxide levels and bispectral index monitoring are the latest advances in monitoring techniques in PSA.

The duration of preprocedural fasting is controversial. The intent of a preprocedural fast is to minimize the risk of pulmonary aspiration. Pulmonary aspiration has yet to be reported for PSA in the emergency department, and its risk in the emergency setting appears to be at best remote. Although the ASA guidelines are not based on evidence, the evaluation and documentation of the last oral intake is a JCAHO requirement. Although the practitioner cannot control the timing of the last oral intake, the depth of sedation and the use of adjunctive techniques such as regional anesthesia can be controlled. When appropriate, high-risk patients should be referred to the operating room for general anesthesia rather then undergoing the risk of emergency department sedation. After PSA, a child must awaken to his or her baseline mental and ambulatory status before being discharged home.

References

[1] Godwin S, Caro D, Wolf S, et al. Clinical policy for procedural sedation and analgesia in the emergency department. Ann Emerg Med 2005;45:177–96.
[2] American Society of Anesthesiologists. Practice guidelines for sedation and analgesia by non-anesthesiologists: an updated report by the American Society of Anesthesiologists Task Force on Sedation and Analgesia by Non-Anesthesiologists. Anesthesiology 2002;96:1004–17.
[3] Innes G, Murphy M, Nijssen-Jordan C, et al. Procedural sedation and analgesia in the emergency department. Canadian consensus guidelines. J Emerg Med 1999;17:145–56.
[4] American Academy of Pediatrics Committee on Drugs. Guidelines for monitoring and management of pediatric patients during and after sedation for diagnostic and therapeutic procedures. Pediatrics 1992;89:110–5.
[5] American Academy of Pediatrics Committee on Drugs. Guidelines for monitoring and management of pediatric patients during and after sedation for diagnostic and therapeutic procedures: addendum. Pediatrics 2002;110:836–8.
[6] Pitetti R, Singh S, Pierce M. Safe and efficacious use of procedural sedation and analgesia by nonanesthesiologists in a pediatric emergency department. Arch Pediatr Adolesc Med 2003; 157:1090–6.
[7] Prstojevich S, Sabol S, Goldwasser M, et al. Utility of capnography in predicting venous carbon dioxide partial pressure in sedated patients during outpatient oral surgery. J Oral Maxillofac Surg 1992;50:37–9.
[8] Iwaski J, Vann Jr W, Dilley D, et al. An investigation of capnography and pulse oximetry as monitors of pediatric patients sedated for dental treatment. Pediatr Dent 1989;11:111–7.
[9] Croswell R, Dilley D, Lucas W, et al. A comparison of conventional versus electronic monitoring of sedated pediatric dental patients. Pediatr Dent 1995;15:332–9.
[10] Yldzdas D, Yapcoglu H, Ylmaz H. The value of capnography during sedation or sedation/analgesia in pediatric minor procedures. Pediatr Emerg Care 2004;20:162–5.
[11] Connor L, Burrows P, Zurakowski D, et al. Effects of IV pentobarbital with and without fentanyl on end-tidal carbon dioxide levels during deep sedation of pediatric patients undergoing MRI. AJR Am J Roentgenol 2003;181:1691–4.

[12] Wright S. Conscious sedation in the emergency department: the value of capnography and pulse oximetry. Ann Emerg Med 1992;21:551–5.

[13] Miner J, Heegaard W, Plummer D. End-tidal carbon dioxide monitoring during procedural sedation. Acad Emerg Med 2002;9:275–80.

[14] Sandler N, Sparks B. The use of bispectral analysis in patients undergoing intravenous sedation for third molar extractions. J Oral Maxillofac Surg 2000;58:364–8.

[15] Overly F, Wright R, Connor F, et al. Bispectral analysis during deep sedation of pediatric oral surgery patients. J Oral Maxillofac Surg 2005;63:215–9.

[16] Bower A, Ripepi A, Dilger J, et al. Bispectral index monitoring of sedation during endoscopy. Gartrointest Endosc 2000;52:192–6.

[17] Powers K, Nazarian E, Tapyrik S, et al. Bispectral index as a guide for titration of propofol during procedural sedation among children. Pediatrics 2005;115:1666–74.

[18] Miner J, Biros M, Heegaard W, et al. Bispectral electroencephalographic analysis of patients undergoing procedural sedation in the emergency department. Acad Emerg Med 2003; 10:638–43.

[19] Miner J, Biros M, Seigel T, et al. The utility of the bispectral index in procedural sedation with propofol in the emergency department. Acad Emerg Med 2005;12:190–6.

[20] Levine D, Platt S. Novel monitoring techniques for use with procedural sedation. Curr Opin Pediatr 2005;17:351–4.

[21] Pershad J, Godambe S. Propofol for procedural sedation in the pediatric emergency department. J Emerg Med 2004;27:11–4.

[22] Kennedy R, Luhmann J, Luhmann S. Emergency department managemen of pain and anxiety related to orthopedic fracture care: a guide to analgesic techniques and procedural sedation in children. Paediatr Drugs 2004;6:11–31.

[23] Parker R, Mahan R, Giugliano D, et al. Efficacy and safety of intravenous midazolam and ketamine as sedation for therapeutic and diagnostic procedures in children. Pediatrics 1997;99: 427–31.

[24] Graff K, Kennedy R, Jaffe D. Conscious sedation for the orthopaedic emergencies. Pediatr Emerg Care 1996;12:31–5.

[25] Guenther E, Pribble C, Junkins Jr E, et al. Propofol sedation by emergency physicians for elective pediatric outpatient procedures. Ann Emerg Med 2003;42:783–91.

[26] Bassett K, Anderson J, Pribble C, et al. Propofol for procedural sedation in the emergency department. Ann Emerg Med 2003;42:773–82.

[27] Pena B, Krauss B. Adverse events of procedural sedation and analgesia in a pediatric emergency department. Ann Emerg Med 1999;34:483–91.

[28] Graff K, Kennedy R, Jaffe D. Conscious sedation for pediatric orthopedic emergencies. Pediatr Emerg Care 1996;12:31–5.

[29] Mace SE, Barata IA, Cravero JP, et al. Clinical policy: evidence-based approach to pharmacologic agents used in pediatric sedation and analgesia in the emergency department. Ann Emerg Med 2004;44(4):342–77.

[30] Cote C, Karl H, Notterman D, et al. Adverse sedation events in pediatrics: analysis of medications used for sedation. Pediatrics 2000;106:633–44.

[31] Green S, Rothrock S, Lynch E, et al. Intramuscular ketamine for pediatric sedation in the emergency department: safety profile in 1,022 cases. Ann Emerg Med 1998;31:688–97.

[32] Sacchetti A, Carraccio C, Giardino A, et al. Sedation for pediatric CT scanning: is radiology becoming a drug-free zone. Pediatr Emerg Care 2005;21:295–7.

[33] Commission on Accreditation of Healthcare Organizations. Accreditation manual for hospitals. St Louis (MO): Mosby-Year Book; 1993.

[34] Malviya S, Voepel-Lewis T, Tait A. Adverse events and risk factors associated with the sedation of children by nonanesthesiologists. Anesth Analg 1997;85:1207–13.

[35] Scarfone R. Sedation and analgesia. In: Selbst SM, Cronan K, editors. Pediatric emergency medicine secrets. Philadelphia: Hanley and Belfus; 2001. p. 385–91.

[36] Mendelson CL. The aspiration of stomach contents into the lungs during obstetric anesthesia. Am J Obstet Gynecol 1946;52:191–205.

[37] Greenfield SM, Webster GJM, Vicary FR. Drinking before sedation. BMJ 1997;314:162.
[38] American Society of Anesthesiologists. Practice guidelines for preoperative fasting and the use of pharmacologic agents to reduce the risk of pulmonary aspiration: applications to healthy patients undergoing elective procedures. Anesthesiology 1999;90:896–905.
[39] Green SM. Fasting is a consideration – not a necessity – for emergency department procedural sedation and analgesia. Ann Emerg Med 2003;42:647–50.
[40] Roback MG, Lalit B, Wathen JE, et al. Preprocedural fasting and adverse events in procedural sedation and analgesia in a pediatric emergency department: are they related? Ann Emerg Med 2004;44:454–9.
[41] Agrawal D, Manzi SF, Gupta R, et al. Preprocedural fasting state and adverse events in children undergoing procedural sedation and analgesia in a pediatric emergency department. Ann Emerg Med 2003;42:636–46.
[42] Greenfield SM, Webster GJM, Vicary FR. Drinking before sedation. BMJ 1997;314:162.
[43] Sutherland AD, Maltby JR, Sale JP, et al. The effect of preoperative oral fluid and ranitidine on gastric fluid volume and pH. Can J Anaesth 1987;34:117–21.
[44] Philips S, Hutchinson S, Davidson T. Preoperative drinking does not affect gastric contents. Br J Anaesth 1993;70:6–9.
[45] Treston G. Prolonged pre-procedure fasting time is unnecessary when using titrated intravenous ketamine for pediatric procedural sedation. Emerg Med Australas 2004;16(2):145–50.
[46] Maltby JR. The shortened fluid fast and the Canadian Anaesthetists's Society's new guidelines for fasting in elective/emergency patients. Can J Anaesth 1990;37:905–6.
[47] Green SM, Krauss B. Pulmonary aspiration risk during emergency department procedural sedation: an examination of the role of fasting and sedation depth. Acad Emerg Med 2002;9:35–42.
[48] Green S, Krauss B. Clinical practice guideline for emergency department ketamine dissociative sedation in children. Ann Emerg Med 2004;44:460–71.

ELSEVIER
SAUNDERS

PEDIATRIC CLINICS
OF NORTH AMERICA

Pediatr Clin N Am 53 (2006) 293–315

Deadly Ingestions

Keith Henry, MD[a], Carson R. Harris, MD[b],*

[a]Emergency Medicine Department, Saint John's Hospital, Maplewood, MN 55109-1169, USA
[b]Emergency Medicine Department, Regions Hospital, 640 Jackson Street, St. Paul, MN 55101, USA

Pediatric patients comprise approximately 52% of the 2.4 million toxic-exposure calls to US Poison Centers [1]. Although most of the cases are minor, the ingestion of at least seven different types of substances can lead to severe toxicity or even death. The 2003 data from the American Association of Poison Control Centers reported 34 deaths in children under the age 6 years, or 3.2% of all fatalities [1]. This was the second highest number of reported deaths in this age group during the 20 years of data collection. The availability of potentially deadly drugs is increasing because of their widespread use in various traditional and newer uses for medical and psychiatric conditions. This availability only serves to increase the likelihood of pediatric encounters and subsequent ingestion. It is therefore important that the clinician be familiar with the presenting signs and symptoms of potentially toxic ingestions and be able to initiate therapeutic and life saving interventions. This article reviews some of the deadlier ingestions to which children may be exposed.

Sulfonylureas

Toxic exposure to oral hypoglycemic drugs continues to increase at a steady rate. Data collected from the 2003 Toxic Exposure Surveillance System (TESS) indicate that well over 10,000 oral hypoglycemic exposures were reported to participating poison control centers. Sulfonylurea agents, considered to be the cornerstone in the treatment of type 2 diabetes, comprised 4019 of the reported

* Corresponding author.
  E-mail address: harri037@umn.edu (C.R. Harris).

0031-3955/06/$ – see front matter © 2006 Elsevier Inc. All rights reserved.
doi:10.1016/j.pcl.2005.09.007

Table 1
Sulfonylureas

	Onset (h)	Duration of action (h)	Half-life (h)
First generation			
Chlorpropamide (Diabinese, 100, 250 mg)	1	24–72	36
Tolazamide (Tolinase, 100, 250, 500 mg)	≤1 (peak 4–6)	16–24	7
Acetohexamide (Dymelor, 250, 500 mg)	1–2	12–24	1.3–1.5 (active metabolite 2–6)
Tolbutamide (Orinase, 500 mg)	1	6–12	7 (4–25)
Second generation			
Glipizide (Glucotrol, 5,10 mg; Glucotrol XL, 5,10 mg)	0.5–3	Up to 24	2–6
Glyburide (Diabeta, Micronase, 1.25, 2.5, 5 mg; Glynase, 1.5, 3, 6 mg)	0.25–1	18–24	1.4–1.8 (metabolite 5–26)
Third generation			
Glimepiride (Amaryl, 1, 2, 4 mg)	1–2	16–30	12–24

Data from Buse JB, Polonsky KS, Burant CS. Type 2 diabetes mellitus. In: Larsen PR, Kronenberg HM, Melmed S, et al, editors. Williams textbook of endocrinology. 10th edition. Philadelphia: WB Saunders; 2003. p. 1427–68.

exposures, with greater than one third occurring in children less than 6 years of age [1].

Table 1 lists the generations of sulfonylureas. The second-generation sulfonylureas (glimepiride, glipizide, and glyburide) exert their action by binding to specific membrane receptors within pancreatic beta islet cells, ultimately causing the inhibition of ATP-dependent potassium channels. As intracellular potassium rises, the cellular membrane depolarizes, allowing for an increase in intracellular calcium from voltage-gated channels and a subsequent release of preformed insulin into the systemic circulation [2,3]. Sulfonylureas will concurrently suppress endogenous glycogenolysis, creating a further potential for symptomatic and life-threatening hypoglycemia [2,4].

Case reports indicate that one or two tablets of a sulfonylurea compound have the potential to cause permanent neurologic disability or death [5,6]. With an increased prevalence of type 2 diabetes transcending all community, cultural, racial, and gender boundaries, the acquisition of sulfonylurea agents represents a clear and present danger to all pediatric populations.

Clinical presentation

Early in the evaluation of the ill or injured child, a thoughtful consideration of toxicologic causes is always appropriate. Sulfonylurea ingestion may present with a broad spectrum of symptoms, from asymptomatic to overt coma and imminent death. Loss of appetite, weakness, dizziness, lethargy, and seizure have all been associated with significant sulfonylurea ingestion [2,4,5,7]. Behavioral changes combined with a suspicion of possible ingestion from a parent, grandparent, friend, or care provider must always prompt a high index of suspicion and careful evaluation. The clinician must always be acutely aware of sulfonylurea ingestion with the potential to present with late symptomatic hypoglycemia. This category includes but is by no means limited to commonly prescribed agents such as chlorpropamide, glyburide, and glucotrol XL [4,5,8].

Management

The management of sulfonylurea ingestion stems largely from data collected and pooled from poison control centers, retrospective reviews, and case studies found within the adult and pediatric toxicology literature [4–10]. Serious pediatric ingestion even at low doses of sulfonylureas has been documented on numerous occasions, leading to the belief that as little as one tablet carries a serious potential for lethality. Considerable controversy exists over the exact time of observation regarding the asymptomatic child who is suspected of having taken an overdose. Based on the authors' experience, a full 24-hour observation period is advocated to allow safe disposition to home with planned follow-up. However, some experts advocate an earlier disposition if the serum glucose level remains above 60 mg/dL for 8 hours [5]. Any documented hypoglycemic episodes or neurologic deteriorations obviously warrant an extension of observation time [4,5,8–10]. During the observation time period, in the absence of documented hypoglycemia or mental status deterioration, oral supplements should be encouraged.

During the initial evaluation, bedside glucose testing and a rapid primary survey of the patient's airway, breathing, and circulation are crucial. A deterioration of the patient's mental status should signal the administration of a weight-based bolus of dextrose, D25, 2 to 4 mL/kg, in children 1 to 24 months of age and D50, 1 to 2 mL/kg in children greater than 24 months, because early intervention is likely to improve mental status quickly, along with any deficiencies encountered during the primary survey.

After the initial evaluation, resuscitation, and stabilization is performed, primary toxicology principals should be applied. Removal of the toxin from the patient may be facilitated partially with the use of activated charcoal, 1g/kg; however, benefits exceeding 1 hour after ingestion are questionable [11]. With the potential for an extended-release preparation to cause delayed hypoglycemia, whole-bowel irrigation has been advocated as an adjunct measure to clear ingested toxin from the patient [12]. However, this measure is considered by many authorities to be lacking in evidence and may pose a significant risk of aspiration [12,13].

Significant sulfonylurea ingestion has been shown in case reports to be refractory to intravenous (IV) boluses of dextrose. In these cases, it is important to consider an IV glucose infusion to maintain a blood glucose level above 60 mg/dL to optimize ample glucose reserves. It is important to remember that continuous glucose infusion may potentiate further insulin release, thereby resulting in breakthrough hypoglycemia episodes [4]. Careful blood glucose monitoring every 1 to 2 hours and frequent neurologic evaluations may indicate the administration of supplemental IV dextrose boluses.

Octreotide has been studied and used as an adjunct to the treatment for sulfonylurea-induced hypoglycemia [14–17] and is recommended currently for serious sulfonylurea toxicity or recalcitrant hypoglycemia [4,5,7,14–17]. Octreotide is a somatostatin analog capable of the direct inhibition of insulin secretion. Its value has been suggested through multiple case reviews and studies; however, evaluation within the pediatric population has been limited. One case report indicates the successful management in a 5-year-old child who presented with profound hypoglycemia and status epilepticus after a glipizide overdose. Treatment included benzodiazepines, dextrose infusion, and octreotide, resulting in seizure cessation, improvement of hypoglycemia, and rapid weaning of glucose infusion [17]. Octreotide should be considered in cases of symptomatic hypoglycemia or in cases of hypoglycemia refractory to initial IV infusions or boluses of dextrose. Published dosing recommendations include 4 to 5 μg/kg/d subcutaneous octreotide given in divided doses every 6 hours to a maximum dose of 50 μg every 6 hours [5].

Glucagon has been used for many years as a therapeutic modality for the treatment of induced hypoglycemia. Glucagon is an endogenous catabolic hormone produced and released from pancreatic alpha cells in the islets of Langerhans. It increases circulating glucose levels by stimulating hepatic glycogenolysis and glycogen breakdown and the induction of gluconeogenesis and ketone production within the liver. When oral glucose replacement is contraindicated and peripheral IV access has proven difficult, intramuscular (IM) administration of glucagon is a viable option [18]. In children, dosing recommendations include giving 0.025 to 0.1 mg/kg, intravenously, subcutaneously, or intramuscularly. The maximum amount per dose recommended is 1 mg. Repeat dosing intervals may proceed every 20 minutes as required. The risk of vomiting and aspiration must be carefully weighed before the administration because glucagon is well known for its emetic response. The clinician must keep in mind that glucagon does not inhibit sulfonylurea-induced insulin release and that hypoglycemia may ultimately persist. Glucagon should be considered as a temporary measure in the emergent treatment of sulfonylurea-induced hypoglycemia.

Calcium channel antagonists

Calcium channel antagonists are used widely in the management of a variety of medical conditions, such as hypertension, angina pectoris, supraventricular dysrhythmias, subarachnoid hemorrhage, and migraine prophylaxis. There are currently ten calcium antagonists on the market in the United States (Table 2). The widespread use and availability of these drugs increase the potential for a child to have access and accidentally ingest one or several of the pills. In 2003, there were 9650 cases of calcium antagonist exposures reported to United States

Table 2
Calcium channel antagonists

Class	Agent	Trade name
Dihydropyridines	Amlodipine	Norvasc
	Felodipine	Plendil
	Nicardipine	Cardene, Cardene SR
	Isradipine	Dynacirc, Dynacirc CR
	Nifedipine	Adalat, Adalat CC, Procardia, Procardia XL
	Nimodipine	Nimotop
	Nisoldipine	Sular
Phenylalkylamine	Verapamil	Calan, Isoptan, Verelan
Benzothiazepine	Diltiazem	Cardizem, Cartia XT, Taztia, Tiazac

poison centers, and approximately 23% of these involved children under the age of 6 years [1].

Clinical presentation

Calcium antagonists block the entry of calcium through voltage-sensitive L-type cellular membrane calcium channels. In vascular tissue, this results in arterial smooth muscle relaxation and hypotension. In cardiac cells, these agents inhibit sinoatrial and atrioventricular nodal depolarization, depress contractility, and cause bradycardia. Insulin release from pancreatic islet cells is inhibited by calcium antagonists and consequently leads to hyperglycemia [19,20]. Lactic acidosis is a common finding and is likely caused by tissue hypoperfusion.

Children can become symptomatic with exposure to as few as one or two tablets, especially in the toddler-aged group [8,19–24]. The ingestion of a single tablet may possibly cause death [24]. The onset of symptoms usually occurs within 1 to 2 hours of ingestion but may be delayed for up to 24 hours with extended-release (extended release [XL], coated tablet with fast release core [CC], controlled release [CR], sustained release [SR]) preparations. A classic presentation of calcium antagonist overdose is bradycardia with hypotension. Other dysrhythmias that may occur include junctional escape rhythms, idioventricular rhythms, atrioventricular (AV) conduction abnormalities, and complete AV block [20]. With the ingestion of dihydropyridine (nifedipine and others), the child may present with hypotension and reflex tachycardia caused by a lack of significant sinoatrial node effect. Tachycardia may occur alone after nifedipine overdose [21]. Typically, conduction abnormalities are rare with dihydropyridine agents because of absent AV node blockade [20].

The child may present with symptoms that include unsteady gait or dizziness, obtundation, coma, and seizure activity [20,21,23] caused by cerebral hypoperfusion. Gastrointestinal symptoms may include nausea and vomiting secondary to diminished gastric motility. Bowel hypoperfusion may cause mesenteric ischemia [21]. Ileus and small bowel obstruction have also been described and may prolong drug absorption and make decontamination efforts challenging [5]. Metabolic features include hyperglycemia and lactic acidosis. Finally, pulmonary edema has also been reported [12,13], resulting from poor myocardial function, but noncardiogenic pulmonary edema has been described as well [14,15].

Management

All children who are suspected of having ingested calcium channel blockers of any amount should be evaluated in a health care facility and monitored in an ICU setting for signs of delayed toxicity. The caretakers should be questioned carefully whenever a child presents with depressed blood pressure or heart rate to determine whether anyone in the household is taking blood pressure or heart medicine.

Treatment of severe hypotension and bradycardia should begin with intravenous fluids, atropine, and calcium chloride. Additional pressor agents may be required, and choices include epinephrine, dopamine, and norepinephrine [25,26]. Atropine is notorious for being ineffective or at least inconsistently effective. More recently, the addition of insulin and glucose, known as hyperinsulinemia euglycemic (HIE) treatment, has gained acceptance as an early intervention in the treatment of toxin-induced shock states [26]. Although the ideal starting regimen for HIE has not been established, a continuous infusion of insulin, 0.5 to 1 unit per kilogram of body weight per hour, has been used to reverse cardiovascular collapse caused by calcium channel blocker overdose. Despite the high doses of insulin administered, some patients may not require supplemental glucose [26,27]. It should be remembered that potassium levels should be checked frequently (at least every hour at the initiation of treatment) and glucose should be monitored closely [28]. It has been suggested that HIE therapy may be considered as a first-line therapy in calcium channel blocker intoxication [25]. Before this therapy can be recommended as the first-line treatment, however, more research is needed.

Glucagon has been used as an adjunct therapy to improve inotropic, chronotropic, and dromotropic effects of calcium antagonist overdose. However, a review of animal models of calcium antagonist poisoning treated with glucagon indicates that glucagon does not improve survival [29]. To date, there are no controlled human clinical trials comparing the effectiveness of glucagon therapy in calcium antagonist overdose.

Toxic alcohols

Toxic alcohols, such as ethanol, isopropanol, methanol, and ethylene glycol (EG), are available in a wide array of commercial and consumer products (Table 3). Ethanol is found in varying concentrations of alcoholic beverages for adults. Because they are ubiquitous substances, these alcohols represent a clear and present danger to the pediatric population. The consequences of even a small ingestion in children carry the potential for death and permanent disability. In 2003, the TESS database reported nearly 84,000 exposures to the alcohol and

Table 3
Toxic alcohol sources

Alcohol	Sources
Ethylene glycol	Radiator antifreeze
	Brake fluid (hydraulic)
	Cellophane softening agent
	Condensers and heat exchangers
	De-icing solutions
	Paints, lacquers, detergents, cosmetics
	Foam stabilizer
	Solvent
Methanol	Windshield wiper fluid
	Industrial solvent
	Gasoline additives, coolants
	Fuel octane booster
	Sterno (picnic stoves, torches)
	Paints and varnishes
	Solvent for extraction (illicit methamphetamine labs)
	Contaminated home-brewed beverages
	Duplicating chemicals
Isopropanol	Rubbing alcohol (70%–91% concentration)
	Industrial solvents
	Paints and paint thinners
	Inks
	Hair tonics

automotive product categories [1]. Ethanol accounted for more than 5600 exposures in patients under the age of 6 years. Isopropanol accounted for approximately 25,000 of the toxic alcohol exposures [1].

Although the parent alcohols can be responsible for a variable degree of central nervous system (CNS) depression, life-threatening conditions are often the result of toxic products resulting from metabolic breakdown, as shown in Table 4 [30]. Alcohols uniformly display rapid absorption profiles from the

Table 4
Toxic alcohols metabolism

Alcohol	Enzyme	Metabolite	Enzyme/cofactor	Metabolite
Isopropyl alcohol	Alcohol dehydrogenase	Acetone[b]		
Methanol	Alcohol dehydrogenase[a]	Formaldehyde	H_2O	Methanediol
	Aldehyde dehydrogenase	Formate[b]		
Ethylene glycol	Alcohol dehydrogenase[a]	Glycoaldehyde	Aldehyde dehydrogenase	Glycolate
	LDH or glycolic acid oxidase[c]	Glyoxylate[b]	B6	→Glycine
			Thiamine, Mg^{2+}	→α-hydroxy-β-ketoadipate
			—	→Oxalate[b]

Abbreviations: B6, pyridoxine; LDH, lactate dehydrogenase.
[a] Rate-limiting step.
[b] Toxic metabolite.
[c] Second rate-limiting step.

gastrointestinal tract, often eliciting signs of intoxication within 30 minutes of ingestion [30]. The metabolism of volatile alcohols occurs through the action of alcohol dehydrogenase (ADH). Further breakdown is achieved through other enzyme systems and pathways and is unique to each specific alcohol. Interventions focus primarily on the competitive inhibition of alcohol dehydrogenase, the enzyme serving as the rate-limiting step in alcohol breakdown [31].

Knowledge of the pharmacokinetics and metabolism of the volatile alcohol group may assist in the recognition and diagnosis of ingestion. Alcohols are of low molecular weight and display osmotically active properties when in solution. These particles are typically absent in serum concentrations and are usually not included in clinical calculations of serum osmolality. The formula for calculating osmolality is 2(Na) + (glucose [mg/dL]) ÷ 18 + (blood urea nitrogen [BUN] [mmol/L]) ÷ 2.8; or, an alternative equation is 1.86(Na) + (BUN) + (glucose) ÷ 0.93.

The difference between the laboratory measurement of osmolality and the calculated osmolarity provides the osmolal gap, or osmolal gap = osm measured − osm calculated. A discrepancy of greater than 10 to 15 mosm/kg H_2O may support the ingestion of a volatile alcohol [31,32]. It cannot be overemphasized, however, that the absence of an osmolar gap does not exclude volatile alcohol ingestion [30,31]. Another useful characteristic of methanol and ethylene glycol ingestion is their potential to cause an anion gap acidosis through the formation of organic acids. In all patients presenting with increased anion gap metabolic acidosis, ethylene glycol or methanol poisoning should be considered, especially in the absence of shock. Isopropanol is converted to nonacidic metabolites and thus does not cause acidosis in the absence of co-ingestions. This characteristic distinguishes isopropanol from ethylene glycol or methanol ingestion and may further assist in the evaluation and diagnosis [30,31]. Volatile alcohol measurements, if available, can rapidly expedite a diagnosis, but awaiting results should never delay treatment.

Clinical presentation

Isopropanol

Isopropanol causes two to three times the intoxicating effect of ethanol at similar serum concentrations. It crosses the blood-brain barrier with particular ease, leading to variable CNS depression, based on the amount of ingestion. The isopropanol metabolite acetone was believed to be the cause of CNS effects, but that remains controversial [33,34]. Respiratory depression, coma, and hypotension are common symptoms with ingestions measuring ≥ 400 mg/dL [35,36]. A child may present with hemorrhagic gastritis and hematemesis if a significant amount has been ingested.

Methanol

Symptoms of methanol ingestion may be delayed for up to 72 hours in some cases [32]. Methanol is well absorbed by inhalation, ingestion, or dermal exposure. It is oxidized in the liver to formaldehyde and then to formic acid, which contributes to the profound metabolic acidosis occurring in acute methanol poisoning. The metabolic products of methanol can produce a syndrome of delayed-onset acidosis, obtundation, visual disturbance, and death. An observed triad of symptoms includes abdominal pain, visual changes, and acidosis. CNS depression and agitation can occur. The metabolite formic acid is extremely lethal, and death has been reported with as little as 15 to 30 mL (1 to 2 tablespoons) of ingested methanol [8,37,38]. Recently, this claim of lethal low-volume ingestion has come under question after a critical review of the literature [39]. Patients may describe visual loss or snowfield vision that occurs typically late in ingestion. Although visual acuity assessment in the toddler may be difficult, attempts should be made to evaluate the fundi as well as vision. Blindness is usually permanent but can be avoided in cases of early presentation, diagnosis, and intervention.

Ethylene glycol

The ingestion of as little as 3 mL of a product containing 95% ethylene glycol carries the potential for lethality in toddler-aged children [8]. Ethylene glycol toxicity often manifests in three different clinical phases. The first phase, occurring up to 12 hours after ingestion, displays altered CNS findings, including decreased mental status, slurred speech, ataxia, hallucinations, coma, and seizures. Cardiopulmonary effects dominate during the second phase and occur 12 to 24 hours after ingestion. Tachycardia, tachypnea, hypertension, congestive heart failure, acute respiratory distress syndrome, and circulatory collapse are encountered commonly at this time. The third and final clinical phase occurs 24 to 72 hours after ingestion and manifests primarily as toxic metabolite-mediated nephrotoxicity [3]. Additionally, the precipitation of calcium into calcium oxalate crystals may cause hypocalcemia, presenting as tetany and prolongation of the QT interval on EKG [40]. Oxalate crystals, which may be found in the child's urine, are more typically the monohydrate type (needle shaped) than the dihydrate (envelope shaped) crystals. Because some ethylene glycol-containing products contain fluorescein, the urine may fluoresce, although this is not a definitive test and cannot be relied on to confirm or refute the diagnosis of ingestion.

Management

Initial laboratory and ancillary tests should include obtaining levels of electrolytes, BUN, creatinine, glucose, lactate, and ionized calcium and an electrocardiogram. In addition, methanol and ethylene glycol levels should be determined, and a urinalysis and arterial blood gas analysis should be performed. A chest radiograph is indicated if there is suspicion that the child may have aspirated or has pulmonary edema. In methanol poisoning, the degree of acidosis and magnitude of the anion gap elevation tend to correlate with blood formate concentrations [30]. In ethylene glycol poisoning, an increased anion gap acidosis correlates with glycolate levels [41]. Seizures may be an indication of hypocalcemia and should be treated with benzodiazepines. For hypoglycemia, give glucose, 50% or 25%, 2 mL/kg body weight in children. Thiamine and pyridoxine are adjunct therapies in EG poisoning, as are folic acid or folinic acid in methanol poisoning (1 mg/kg, or up to 50 mg). Symptomatic hypocalcemia should be treated using calcium gluconate. Calcium should not be given for hypocalcemia alone because it may increase the formation of calcium oxalate crystals [37].

Isopropanol

Airway protection is paramount, and the clinician should maintain a low threshold for intubation and mechanical ventilation. Hypotension will usually respond to a fluid bolus. Hemodialysis, although rarely indicated, may greatly enhance serum elimination and is considered definitive management in cases of prolonged coma and hypotension [36].

Methanol and ethylene glycol

The cornerstone of management includes the correction of acidosis, competitive inhibition of ADH, and hemodialysis-assisted elimination. The antidote fomepizole acts through the binding of ADH 500 to 1000 times more effectively than methanol, essentially eliminating the formation of toxic metabolites. For methanol poisoning, this antidote is indicated with symptomatic toxicity, methanol levels ≥ 20 mg/dL or pH level ≤ 7.20 [37–40,42]. A loading dose of 15 mg/kg is given initially, followed by 10 mg/kg every 12 hours for 48 hours and then 15 mg/kg until the methanol level is below 20 mg/dL [43,44].

Historically, a 10% ethanol solution has been used to elicit competitive inhibition of toxic metabolizes. When fomepizole is not available, oral or IV ethanol is the antidote of choice, along with other adjunctive care. Serum ethanol concentrations should be maintained between 100 and 150 mg/dL. Dosing schedules are variable, and the clinician must be aware of the potential risk for aspiration and further CNS decline [37]. Most authorities ascribe an overall cost savings with the use of fomepizole; however, ethanol still exists as a viable option [40].

Hemodialysis is considered a definitive treatment modality and should be considered early in cases suspected of having methanol or ethylene glycol ingestion. Indications include visual impairment, profound acidosis, renal failure, and methanol or ethylene glycol values greater than 50 mg/dL (Table 5) [40,43]. In methanol poisoning, folate should be given at a dose of 1 mg/kg intravenously in 100 mL D5W over 30 to 60 minutes, up to 50 mg every 4 hours for six doses [45]. This treatment serves as an enzyme cofactor in the conversion of formate to CO_2 and water [37,45]. Most authorities suggest ICU admission for close observation during the early stages of therapy. In cases of EG poisoning, pyridoxine and thiamine should be given daily because they will help shunt the toxic metabolite glyoxalate through nontoxic pathways. Cardiac monitoring in the

Table 5
Indications for hemodialysis in toxic alcohol poisoning

Treatment	Dose	Indication
Fomepizole	15 mg/kg loading dose, followed by 10 mg/kg q12 h for 48 h, then 15 mg/kg q12 h until toxic alcohol level ≤20 mg/dL	Ingestion of multiple substances with depressed level of consciousness Altered consciousness Inability to provide intensive care staffing or monitor ethanol administration Relative contraindication to ethanol Critically ill patient with an anion gap metabolic acidosis of unknown cause and potential exposure to ethylene glycol or methanol Patients with active hepatic disease
Ethanol (10%)	600–800 mg/kg (0.6–0.8 g/kg or 6–8 mL/kg) loading dose, then 0.83 mL/kg/h maintenance: monitor serum ethanol level q1–2 h to maintain level 100–150 mg/dL	Unable to give fomepizole Able to provide adequate intensive care staffing and obtain ethanol levels in timely manner Strong clinical suspicion of toxic alcohol ingestion and metabolic acidosis with osmolal gap ≥10 mosm/kg H_2O
Hemodialysis		Severe metabolic acidosis (pH 7.25–7.3) unresponsive to therapy Renal failure (Cr ≥3.0) EG or methanol level ≥50 mg/dL unless fomepizole is being administered and patient is asymptomatic with normal arterial pH

Data from Casavant MJ. Fomepizole in the treatment of poisoning. Pediatrics 2001;107(1):170–1.

pediatric ICU is always appropriate because of the potential for cardiopulmonary decline.

Clonidine

Clonidine is a commonly prescribed, centrally acting antihypertensive, which recently has enjoyed an expanded therapeutic role in the treatment of pediatric attention deficit hyperactivity disorder and Tourette's syndrome. Clonidine is a central α-adrenoreceptor agonist that allows inhibition of sympathetic outflow. Because of its widespread use in all age populations, clonidine remains a common substance of pediatric ingestion. In 2002, the TESS reported over 1600 (31%) ingestions in children under the age of 6 years [46]; and in 2003, 5402 clonidine exposures occurred, with 1736 (32%) exposures in children under the age of 6 years [1]. Lethality is attributed largely to toxic effects on the CNS and cardiovascular systems and may be seen with doses as small as 10 μg/kg. The typical exposure scenario is the child who ingests the drug while visiting grandparents, where tablets have been left out on the nightstand or in a loosely capped pill container, which allow easy access for the child.

Clinical presentation

Because of a functional overlap in the α_2 receptors targeted by clonidine and the μ receptors targeted by opioids, the constellation of symptoms that have been described with clonidine toxicity largely resemble an opioid toxidrome [47,48]. Symptoms include altered mental status, somnolence, respiratory depression, miosis, bradycardia, and hypotension. Dose-related responses have been documented, with cardiovascular effects seen with ingestions between 0.01 and 0.02 mg/kg and respiratory depression occurring with ingestions greater that 20 µg/kg [47,49]. Apnea and respiratory depression are common when the dose exceeds 0.02 mg/kg [49]. Most children will have signs or symptoms of toxicity within 30 to 90 minutes after ingestion [47]. The toddler may respond somewhat differently than older children, presenting in a deeply comatose state, with apnea and bradycardia. However when stimulated, the toddler may respond with increased respiration and pulse, with an improved level of consciousness. If the child is not stimulated, she may quickly return to the previous state or even slip into cardiopulmonary arrest [47]. Although they are rare, seizures can occur with significant overdoses.

Management

The management of suspected clonidine overdose remains largely supportive. Careful attention must be focused on the establishment and maintenance of a patent airway. Because of the risks of bradycardia, heart block, and hypotension, continuous cardiac monitoring and a 12-lead EKG should be used. Activated charcoal should be administered if the patient presents within 1 hour of ingestion. The rapid absorption profile of clonidine precludes recommendations for multiple dosing of charcoal [47].

Naloxone has been used with variable success in treating severe clonidine overdose. It has been shown to reverse both cardiovascular and respiratory depression in up to 50% of case reports [47,50–54]. This is likely caused by opioid receptor overlap, as described above. Suggested naloxone dosing is 0.1 mg, up to a maximum of 10 mg [47,52,54]. Refractory cases of bradycardia will usually respond to atropine. Hypotension should be managed with aggressive fluid resuscitation. Dopamine is recommended by most authorities as the vasopressor of choice, starting at 5 µg/kg/min and increasing in 5-µg/kg/min increments as needed. Norepinephrine should be added if more than 20 µg/kg/min of dopamine is needed. At moderate doses, dopamine may provide sufficient blood pressure support, while its chronotropic properties may mitigate clonidine-induced bradycardia [47].

Admission to the pediatric ICU is always appropriate in patients who manifest altered mental status, respiratory depression, or cardiac abnormality. Patients who do not show signs of toxicity within 6 to 8 hours after ingestion are usually safe for discharge after a 6- to 8-hour observation period [50,55–57].

Tricyclic antidepressants

Antidepressant medications are responsible for a large number of ingestion-related deaths each year. According to the 2003 TESS report, tricyclic antidepressants (TCA) are the third leading cause of death after analgesics and sedative-hypnotics and antipsychotics categories [1]. There were over 12,700 reported exposures to tricyclic antidepressants, and over 1500 exposures occurred in children under the age of 6 years. Amitriptyline, imipramine, and nortriptyline comprise the majority of tricyclic ingestions in children less than 6 years of age, accounting for 13% of all prescribed cyclic antidepressants within the last 10 years, in light of the fact that this group of agents is considered a second- and third-line therapy for depression [58]. The acquisition of this medication class is further enhanced because of its expanded therapeutic value. Currently, tricyclic antidepressants are used to treat numerous medical and psychiatric conditions in both adult and pediatric populations [59].

A growing body of evidence suggests that tricyclic antidepressants exert their therapeutic effects through the centrally mediated inhibition of biogenic amines (serotonin and norepinephrine), thereby correcting a theoretical "imbalance" that may manifest initially as psychiatric illness [58,60]. Clinically important peripheral manifestations of TCA use and toxicity include the inhibition of histamine H_1 and muscarinic cholinergic M_1 receptors, the clinical findings of which are discussed below. The hallmark of TCA toxicity is the dangerous blockade of fast voltage-gated sodium channels found on cardiac myocytes. The altered sodium influx effectively slows phase-zero depolarization, manifesting as a widened QRS complex on the EKG; this is an ominous sign in light of a known or suspected TCA ingestion [8,58,60–63].

Clinical presentation

Most authorities agree that TCA doses as low as 15 mg/kg can be lethal among toddler-aged children [61]. Exposures of 5 mg/kg or less are generally well tolerated and may follow an asymptomatic course [58,60,61]. Although the deleterious effects of TCA toxicity are primarily associated with the cardiovascular and central nervous systems, early toxicity may present with signs and symptoms consistent with an anticholinergic toxidrome. Effects on the CNS and peripheral cholinergic receptors may manifest as confusion, delirium, dilated pupils, dry mouth, urinary incontinence, diminished bowel activity, and tachycardia [8,58,60,61]. Mortality, however, is attributed to overt cardiovascular collapse and CNS toxicity, to include seizure and coma.

In the pediatric population, EKG findings can be suggestive and aid in the conformation of TCA toxicity. However, the EKG is unable to provide any prognostic information regarding the severity or outcome of a TCA overdose. EKG findings include sinus tachycardia, ventricular dysrhythmias, heart block, widening QRS and QTc intervals, and an R wave greater than 3 mm in lead aV_R [8,58,60–63].

Management

The management of TCA overdose requires the rapid suspicion or recognition of the offending agent along with aggressive airway and hemodynamic support. Neurologic deterioration and cardiovascular collapse must be anticipated, and aggressive supportive care must be provided. The child may show a sudden change in sensorium, such as sudden seizure or coma. Continuous cardiac monitors, ample IV access, and supplemental oxygen should be employed immediately. Because of its anticholinergic properties, TCA ingestion may cause delayed gastric emptying [8,58,61]. It is therefore essential that activated charcoal be administered as soon as possible in an attempt to minimize further absorption [64].

Neurologic decline occurs quickly with life-threatening amounts of TCA ingestion. Should this occur or appear imminent, intubation and mechanical ventilation is strongly suggested. Seizures are usually responsive to benzodiazepines [8,58]. Barbiturates should be avoided for the risk of potentiating hypotension [8,60]. Phenytoin has been shown to induce ventricular dysrhythmias in animal models, and its use is not recommended to achieve seizure control [58].

Sodium bicarbonate has long been the primary treatment of TCA-induced cardiotoxicity. Some controversy exists over the exact mechanism through which sodium bicarbonate exerts its therapeutic effect. Some animal studies suggest that sodium bicarbonate mitigates toxicity through an increase in serum pH level, whereas others site an increase in serum sodium level [60]. Regardless of the mechanism, sodium bicarbonate is indicated in the event of severe clinical toxicity, widening of the QRS complex ≥ 100 ms, ventricular dysrhythmias, and hypotension [58–63,65,66]. Although drip- versus bolus-dosing strategies remain controversial, a starting IV bolus of 1 to 2 mEq/kg in children is appropriate [8,58,60]. A serum pH level of greater than 7.5 should not be exceeded. The patient must be monitored for the development of hypokalemia, and IV supplementation may be required.

The use of classes IA and IC antidysrhythmics should be strictly avoided based on their potential to exacerbate TCA-induced cardiotoxicity [58,60]. Dopamine and norepinephrine have been used to overcome alpha blockade-induced hypotension. There is no clear evidence to suggest one over the other at this time [60]. The use of physostigmine should be avoided because it may lead to seizures and fatal cardiac dysrhythmias [60].

In cases of accidental ingestion in a child who is asymptomatic, she may be observed in the emergency department (ED) for 6 hours after ingestion. If no evidence of toxicity occurs, the child may be safely discharged in the care of responsible adults. If symptoms do occur during the period of observation in the

ED, appropriate treatment should be initiated, and the child should be admitted to a monitored inpatient setting.

Salicylates

Data from the American Association of Poison Control Centers' annual report for 2003 [1] list the most common classes of substances involved in fatalities as the analgesics, stimulants, street drugs, antidepressants, cardiovascular agents, and sedative-hypnotics-antipsychotics. During this reporting period, an analgesic was believed to be the primary responsible agent in 375 fatalities. Of these, 23 fatalities involved aspirin alone. Over 50% of these patients had salicylate concentrations less than 100 mg/dL. Of the 916 nonaspirin salicylate exposures, 456 involved children less than 6 years of age.

Salicylates can be found in high concentration in several products commonly used in the home and accessible to children; most notably, oil of wintergreen (methyl salicylate), which is contained in liniments or analgesic balms. This product is deceptively toxic, and 1 mL of a 98% concentration is equivalent to 1400 mg of salicylate. Because the toxic dose of salicylate is 200 mg/kg, it is obvious that exposure to less than 1 teaspoonful can be lethal to a toddler. The liquid preparations undergo rapid absorption, typically within 1 hour, and are converted quickly to salicylate [67]. It should be remembered that Chinese herbal medications or Chinese medicated oils may also contain salicylates [68–70]. At toxic doses in children, the elimination half-life of salicylates increases from 2 to 4 hours at therapeutic levels to 15 to 29 hours [71].

Salicylates have several pathophysiologic mechanisms leading to toxicity. Stimulation of the respiratory center in the brainstem causes hyperventilation, with increases in the depth and rate of breathing. The uncoupling of oxidative phosphorylation results in increased oxygen consumption, further respiratory stimulation, metabolic acidosis, and a compensatory response by the kidney to excrete bicarbonate, potassium, and sodium. An increase in pulmonary vascular permeability and an increase in leukotrienes can lead to pulmonary edema [67]. Salicylates toxicity increases glucose consumption, inhibits gluconeogenesis, and enhances insulin secretion [67,72]. These toxic actions can lead to significant hypoglycemia, particularly in children [72] compared with adults.

Clinical presentation

Children under the age of 2 years have a tendency to present with metabolic acidosis, compared with adolescents and adults, who may present with respiratory alkalosis [73]. The child may present with the odor of oil of wintergreen on her breath, lethargy, diaphoresis, and an increase in all vital signs. Severe toxicity may cause coma, seizures, and cardiovascular collapse. Table 6 shows the clinical manifestations of salicylate toxicity. Dehydration is a common presentation secondary to vomiting and the inability to tolerate oral fluids as well

Table 6
Clinical presentation of salicylate toxicity

System	Clinical findings
CNS	Disorientation, combative or agitated
	Hallucinations (auditory)
	Coma, convulsions due to cerebral edema or low cerebrospinal fluid glucose
Gastrointestinal	Nausea, vomiting, and epigastric discomfort
Cardiovascular	Sinus tachycardia, hypotension, ventricular dysrhythmias, shock, asystole
Respiratory	Pulmonary edema, hyperpnea
Renal/acid-base	Renal failure, respiratory alkalosis, mixed respiratory alkalosis, increased anion gap metabolic acidosis
Electrolytes	Dehydration, hypokalemia, hyponatremia or hypernatremia
	Hypoglycemia/hyperglycemia, hypocalcemia/hypercalcemia
Miscellaneous	Tinnitus and deafness, sweating, hyperpyrexia, leukocytosis, hypoprothrombinemia, rhabdomyolysis

as tachypnea, diaphoresis, and early diuresis. Potassium losses from gastro-intestinal and urinary losses, as well as an obligatory intracellular shift of potassium in exchange for hydrogen ions, lead to severe hypokalemia. Of note, clinical deterioration can be rapid, and aggressive management of the sick child is warranted.

Management

Laboratory testing should include a salicylate level, but this level should not be relied on to predict prognosis. The Done nomogram is no longer recommended to assist in predicting the severity of toxicity [74]. The child's clinical presentation coupled with metabolic status should weigh heavily in the treatment and monitoring plan. Arterial blood gases, electrolytes, and serum glucose levels should be carefully monitored and managed appropriately. In the euglycemic patient who has depressed level of consciousness, the management includes monitoring calcium levels because both hypocalcemia and hypercalcemia have been reported in severe salicylate toxicity [75,76].

The administration of oral activated charcoal should be given early after ingestion. Because one of the primary symptoms of this deadly ingestion is vomiting and altered mentation, the child is at risk of aspiration, and appropriate precautions must be instituted. The child may easily present with severe dehydration and require aggressive rehydration. The child's fluid status must be monitored closely in order not to overload the cardiopulmonary system. This should be done in the pediatric ICU setting. Maintaining a urine output of 2 to 3 mL/kg/h is recommended.

After rehydration, another important management goal is to alkalinize the urine to a pH level of 7.5 to 8.5 to enhance the elimination of the salicylate ion. Equally important is to alkalinize the blood to a pH level of 7.5 to 7.55 [72]. One approach to achieving urinary alkalinization is to add 150 mL of sodium bicarbonate to 850 mL of D5W and infuse at a rate of 1.5 to 2 times the maintenance calculated for the child [67]. Alternatively, in a child, sodium bicarbonate may be administered, 25 to 50 mmol (25 mL of an 8.4% solution), intravenously over 1 hour and give additional boluses intravenously to maintain the urine pH level in the range of 7.5 to 8.5. The endpoint of alkalinization is when the salicylate level is less than 25 mg/dL [77].

Most fatal cases of salicylate poisoning are those that fail to receive hemodialysis in a timely manner, which suggests that more aggressive and earlier use of dialysis may be indicated in the treatment of highly concentrated salicylate ingestions. Children who present with or develop significant neurologic presentations (agitation, lethargy, coma, and convulsions), cardiac instability, and renal failure or have significantly elevated or increasing salicylate levels are candidates for hemodialysis. Specific levels should not dictate whether the patient receives hemodialysis, but rather clinical symptoms in conjunction with the level should be considered. Traditionally, levels of 80 to 100 mg/dL were cause for mandatory dialysis. Hemodialysis can also correct the acid-base abnormalities.

Some of the pitfalls in the management of methyl salicylate poisoning are underestimating the toxicity of small amounts, attempting to use the Done nomogram, focusing on urine alkalinization rather than considering blood pH level, hypoventilating the intubated child, which allows the blood pH level to decrease, failing to monitor the patient for hypoglycemia, and failing to initiate hemodialysis when it is clinically indicated [72].

Opioids

Opioids are a popular analgesic for moderate to severe pain. They are also used as adjuncts to anesthesia, cough suppressants, and antidiarrheals. Methadone, a long-acting synthetic narcotic analgesic used in the detoxification treatment of opiate dependence and for maintenance in heroin and narcotic addiction, may also be prescribed for the relief of moderate to severe pain. Opioids can be used recreationally and abused for their sedative and analgesic effects. Because of their widespread use, either legally or illicitly, their availability is high, and children may have easy access to these dangerous agents in the home. The 2003 TESS database reported 34 deaths of children under the age of 6 years. Nine of these fatalities were unintentional general, with six deaths involving prescription medications. Three of the prescription medications were opioids. Overall, of the 375 fatalities implicating analgesic drugs as the primary causative agent of death, 100 involved an acetaminophen-combined product, usually containing an opioid [1].

Although the number of deaths related to methadone or oxycodone compared with 2002 data has decreased, these agents continue to be incriminated to a significant degree in major toxicity. Although the minimal lethal pediatric dose is unknown, a small child who ingests even residual amounts of a methadone suspension left in a bottle can progress from drowsiness to coma within 30 minutes [78]. The increasing use of methadone in the treatment of heroin addiction has created a situation in which the drug may be readily available to children and other family members of maintenance patients, causing serious consequences. Because of their increased mobility after infancy, curiosity, and oral fixation, toddlers may be especially susceptible to getting into illicit narcotics, such as powdered heroin and fentanyl patches, left unattended by the adult. Fentanyl transmucosal lozenges have been reported as the cause of an unintentional death in an 11-year-old child [1].

Opioids interact with three main receptors (μ, κ, and δ) located throughout the CNS and peripheral nervous systems and in the gastrointestinal tract. Activation of these receptors by the opioids results in a variety of life-threatening complications [79].

Clinical presentation

The classic triad of miosis, CNS depression, and respiratory depression should alert the clinician to probable opioid toxicity. Other signs and symptoms of opioid toxicity include dizziness, euphoria or dysphoria, depressed reflexes, altered sensory perception, lethargy, and coma. The child may also display analgesia to painful stimuli, dry mucous membranes, facial flushing, diaphoresis or clammy skin, nausea and vomiting, muscle flaccidity, bronchospasm, and bradycardia [79,80]. Apnea, noncardiogenic pulmonary edema, circulatory collapse, coma, cardiac arrest, and possible death can occur in significant ingestions that go unrecognized or when the child is found too late for effective treatment. It is important to question the adult caretaker regarding the possibility of access to either short- or long-acting narcotics when the child presents with a narcotic syndrome.

Management

The mainstay of treatment for opioid toxicity is the administration of naloxone. The usual initial dose of naloxone for patients with CNS depression without respiratory depression is 0.1 to 0.4 mg intravenously for both adults and children. If there is partial or absent response, then naloxone, 2 mg, should be administered as an intravenous bolus and repeated every 3 minutes up to a total dose of 10 to 20 mg. When there is respiratory depression, initial higher doses of naloxone should be given, starting with 1 to 2 mg. The effective dose may need to be repeated every 20 to 60 minutes, depending on the half-life of the opioid ingested and the patient's response. A continuous infusion is titrated to the patient's respiratory status and level of conscious if long-acting narcotics such as methadone are ingested [79,81]. The infusion rate may be started at two thirds the amount needed to reverse the child's respiratory depression per hour [80].

If an IV is not available, naloxone can be given through almost any route, including intranasally and by nebulizer [82,83]. Although the intranasal route is not as effective as the intramuscular route, it is still effective in reversing opiate-induced respiratory depression [82].

The long-acting narcotic antagonist nalmefene is an option in children who are nonopioid-dependent and not at risk of withdrawal. Although there is limited literature on this treatment in children, it appears to be safe and effective in treating opioid toxicity [84]. If the child presents within 1 hour of ingesting a delayed-absorption product such as diphenoxylate-atropine (Lomotil) or sustained release morphine or oxycodone, activated charcoal should be administered, paying close attention to the mental status and respiratory depression [64]. Activated charcoal should be given at a dose of 1 g/kg, orally or by naso- or orogastric tube.

The decision to discharge, observe in the ED, or admit the patient is still controversial. Children with recurrent respiratory depression after initial treatment with naloxone, who have evidence of pulmonary edema or who have ingested long-acting or delayed absorption opioids, should be admitted. Long-acting opioids such as methadone have a tendency to cause a significant recurrence of symptoms, typically within 2 hours of presentation [85]. Also, consideration of the home environment and safety of the child must be weighed in the decision to release or admit the child.

Summary

The mantra of toxicology is that "the dose makes the poison," and in the case of pediatric ingestions, this is very true. There are scores of products and agents that can be deadly if the appropriate "dose" is ingested. This article presents only a few of the potentially deadly ingestions this patient population might encounter, but the clinician is cautioned to use sound judgment in managing children presenting with a history of being found with pills in their possession. In addition, social issues surrounding the ingestion should be considered when making a disposition.

References

[1] Watson WA, Litovitz TL, Klein-Schwartz W, et al. 2003 Annual report of the American Association of Poison Control Centers Toxic Exposure Surveillance System. Am J Emerg Med 2004;22(5):335–404.
[2] Buse JB, Polonsky KS, Burant CF. Type 2 diabetes mellitus. In: Larsen PR, Kronenberg HM, Melmed S, et al, editors. Williams textbook of endocrinology. 10th edition. Philadelphia: WB Saunders; 2003. p. 1427–68.
[3] Riddle MC. Glycemic management of type 2 diabetes: an emerging strategy with oral agents, insulins, and combinations. Endocrinol Metab Clin North Am 2005;34(1):77–98.
[4] Wolf LR, Smeeks F, Policastro M. Oral hypoglycemic agents. In: Ford MD, Delaney KA, Ling LJ, et al, editors. Clinical toxicology. 1st edition. Philadelphia: WB Saunders; 2001. p. 423–32.
[5] Little G, Boniface K. Are one or two dangerous? sulfonylurea exposure in toddlers. J Emerg Med 2005;28(3):305–10.
[6] Szlatenyi CS, Capers KF, Wang RY. Delayed hypoglycemia in a child after ingestion of a single glipizide tablet. Ann Emerg Med 1998;31(6):773–6.

[7] Spiller HA. Prospective multicenter study of sulfonylurea ingestion in children. J Pediatr 1997; 131:68–78.

[8] Michael J, Sztajnkrycer M. Deadly pediatric poisons: nine common agents that kill at low doses. Emerg Med Clin North Am 2004;22:1019–50.

[9] Borowski H. Sulfonylurea ingestion in children: is an 8 hour observation period sufficient? J Pediatr 1998;133(4):484–5.

[10] Burkhart KK. When does hypoglycemia develop after sulfonylurea ingestion? Ann Emerg Med 1998;31(6):771–2.

[11] Chyka PA, Seger D. Position statement: single-dose activated charcoal. J Toxicol Clin Toxicol 1997;35:721–41.

[12] Tenenbein M. Position statement: whole bowel irrigation. J Toxicol Clin Toxicol 1997;35: 753–62.

[13] Seger D, Meulenbelt J, L'heureux P. Position paper: whole bowel irrigation. J Toxicol Clin Toxicol 2004;42(6):843–55.

[14] McLaughlin SA, Crandall CS, McKinney PE. Octreotide: an antidote for sulfonylurea-induced hypoglycemia. Ann Emerg Med 2000;36(2):133–8.

[15] Spiller HA. Management of sulfonylurea ingestions. Pediatr Emerg Care 1999;15(3):227–30.

[16] Boyle PJ, Justice K, Krentz AJ, et al. Octreotide reverses hyperinsulinemia and prevents hypoglycemia induced by sulfonylurea overdoses. J Clin Endocrinol Metab 1993;76:752–6.

[17] Mordel A, Sivilotti MLA, Old AC, et al. Octreotide for pediatric sulfonylurea poisoning [abstract]. J Toxicol Clin Toxicol 1998;36:437.

[18] Pollack CV. Utility of glucagon in the emergency department. J Emerg Med 1993;11:195–205.

[19] Bar-Oz B, Levichek Z, Koren G. Medications that can be fatal for a toddler with one tablet or teaspoonful: a 2004 update. Paediatr Drugs 2004;6(2):123–6.

[20] Anderson AC. Calcium channel blockers overdose. Clin Ped Emerg Med 2005;6:109–15.

[21] Ramoska EA, Spiller HA, Myers A. Calcium channel blocker toxicity. Ann Emerg Med 1990; 19(6):649–53.

[22] Brayer AF, Wax P. Accidental ingestion of sustained release calcium channel blockers in children. Vet Hum Toxicol 1998;40(2):104–6.

[23] Lee DC, Greene T, Dougherty T, et al. Fatal nifedipine ingestions in children. J Emerg Med 2000;19(4):359–61.

[24] Spiller HA, Romoska EA. Isradipine ingestion in a two-year-old child. Vet Hum Toxicol 1993; 35(3):233.

[25] Rasmussen L, Husted SE, Johnsen SP. Severe intoxication after an intentional overdose of amlodipine. Acta Anaesthesiol Scand 2003;47(8):1038–40.

[26] Boyer EW, Shannon M. Treatment of calcium channel blocker intoxication with insulin infusion. N Engl J Med 2001;344(22):1721–2.

[27] Yuan TH, Kerns II WP, Toamszewski CA, et al. Insulin-glucose a adjunctive therapy for severe calcium channel antagonist poisoning. J Toxicol Clin Toxicol 1999;37(4):463–74.

[28] Boyer EW, Duic PA, Evans A. Hyperinsulinemia/euglycemia therapy for calcium channel blocker poisoning. Pediatr Emerg Care 2002;18:36–7.

[29] Bailey B. Glucagon in beta-blocker and calcium channel blocker overdoses: a systematic review. J Toxicol Clin Toxicol 2003;41:595–602.

[30] Ford MD, McMartin K. Ethylene glycol and methanol. In: Ford MD, Delaney KA, Ling LJ, et al, editors. Clinical toxicology. 1st edition. Philadelphia: WB Saunders; 2001. p. 757–67.

[31] Sharma AN. Toxic alcohols. In: Goldfrank LR, Flomenbaum NE, Lewin NA, et al, editors. Goldfrank's toxicologic emergencies. 7th edition. New York: McGraw-Hill; 2002. p. 980–1003.

[32] Barceloux DG, Bond GR, Krenzelok EP, et al. American Academy of Clinical Toxicology practice guidelines on the treatment of methanol poisoning. J Toxicol Clin Toxicol 2002;40: 415–46.

[33] Gaudet MP, Fraser GL. Isopropanol ingestion: case report with pharmacokinetic analysis. Am J Emerg Med 1989;7:297–9.

[34] Mydler TT, Wasserman GS, Watson WA, et al. Two-week-old infant with isopropanol intoxication. Pediatr Emerg Care 1993;9:146–8.

[35] Burkhart KK, Kulig KW. The other alcohols: methanol, ethylene glycol, and isopropanol. Emerg Med Clin North Am 1990;8(4):913–28.

[36] Ford MD. Isopropanol. In: Ford MD, Delaney KA, Ling LJ, et al, editors. Clinical toxicology. 1st edition. Philadelphia: WB Saunders; 2001. p. 769–73.

[37] Erickson TB, Brent J. Toxic alcohols. In: Erickson TB, Aherns WR, Aks SE, et al, editors. Pediatric toxicology: diagnosis and management of the poisoned child. New York: McGraw-Hill; 2005. p. 326–32.

[38] Bennett IL, Cary FH, Mitchell GL, et al. Acute methyl alcohol poisoning: a review based on experiences in an outbreak of 323 cases. Medicine 1953;32:431–3.

[39] Kostic MA, Dart RC. Rethinking the toxic methanol level. J Toxicol Clin Toxicol 2003;41(6): 793–800.

[40] Barceloux DG, Bond GR, Krenzelok EP, et al. American Academy of Clinical Toxicology practice guidelines on the treatment of methanol poisoning. J Toxicol Clin Toxicol 2002;40(4): 415–46.

[41] Moreau CL, Kerns II W, Tomaszewsi CA, et al. Glycolate kinetics and hemodialysis clearance in ethylene glycol poisoning. J Toxicol Clin Toxicol 1998;36(7):659–66.

[42] Casavant MJ. Fomepizole in the treatment of poisoning. Pediatrics 2001;107(1):170–1.

[43] Barceloux DG, Krenzelok EP, Olson K, et al. American Academy of Clinical Toxicology practice guidelines on the treatment of ethylene glycol poisoning. J Toxicol Clin Toxicol 1999; 37(5):537–60.

[44] Brent J, McMartin K, Phillips S, et al. Fomepizole for the treatment of ethylene glycol poisoning. N Engl J Med 1999;340(11):832–8.

[45] Thomson MicroMedex. Methanol. In: MICROMEDEX Healthcare Series, vol. 125 [expires September 2005].

[46] Watson WA, Litovitz TL, Rodgers Jr GC, et al. 2002 annual report of the American Association of Poison Control Centers Toxic Exposure Surveillance System. Am J Emerg Med 2003;21(5): 353–421.

[47] Henretig FM. Clonidine and central-acting antihypertensives. In: Ford MD, Delaney KA, Ling LJ, et al, editors. Clinical toxicology. 1st edition. Philadelphia: WB Saunders; 2001. p. 391–6.

[48] Kuhar MJ. Receptors for clonidine in brain: insights into therapeutic actions. J Clin Psychiatry 1982;43(6 Pt 2):17–9.

[49] Fiser DH, Moss MM, Walker W. Critical care for clonidine poisoning in toddlers. Crit Care Med 1990;18(10):1124–8.

[50] Bizovi K. Antihypertensives, β-blockers, and calcium antagonists. In: Erickson TB, Aherns WR, Aks SE, et al, editors. Pediatric toxicology: diagnosis and management of the poisoned child. New York: McGraw-Hill; 2005. p. 245–52.

[51] Klein-Schwartz W. Trends and toxic effects from pediatric clonidine exposure. Arch Pediatr Adolesc Med 2002;156:392–6.

[52] Tenenbein M. Naloxone in clonidine toxicity. Am J Dis Child 1984;138:1084.

[53] Abbruzzi G, Stork C. Pediatric toxicologic concerns. Emerg Med Clin North Am 2002;20(1): 223–46.

[54] Wiley JF, Wiley CC, Torrey SB, et al. Clonidine poisoning in young children. J Pediatr 1990; 116(4):654–8.

[55] Kappagoda C, Schell DN, Hanson RM, et al. Clonidine overdose in childhood: implications of increased prescribing. J Paediatr Child Health 1998;34(6):508–12.

[56] Spiller S, Klein-Schwartz W, Colvin J, et al. Toxic clonidine ingestion in children. J Pediatr 2005;146(2):263–6.

[57] Eddy O, Howell JM. Are one or two dangerous? clonidine and topical imidazolines exposure in toddlers. J Emerg Med 2004;27(3):313–4.

[58] Liebelt EL, Francis PD. Tricyclic Antidepressants. In: Goldfrank LR, Flomenbaum NE, Lewin NA, et al, editors. Goldfrank's toxicologic emergencies. 7th edition. New York: McGraw-Hill; 2002. p. 847–64.

[59] Geller B, Reising D, Leonard HL, et al. Critical review of tricyclic antidepressant use in children and adolescents. J Am Acad Child Adolesc Psychiatry 1999;38(5):513–6.

[60] Pentel PR, Keyler DE. Cyclic antidepressants. In: Ford MD, Delaney KA, Ling LJ, et al, editors. Clinical toxicology. 1st edition. Philadelphia: WB Saunders; 2001. p. 515–21.

[61] Rosenbaum T, Kou M. Are one or two dangerous? tricyclic antidepressant exposure in toddlers. J Emerg Med 2005;28(2):169–74.

[62] Liebelt EL, Francis PD, Woolf AD. ECG lead aVR versus QRS interval in predicting seizures and arrhythmias in acute tricyclic antidepressant toxicity. Ann Emerg Med 1995;26(2): 195–201.

[63] Liebelt EL, Ulrich A, Francis PD, et al. Serial electrocardiogram changes in acute tricyclic antidepressant overdoses. Crit Care Med 1997;25:1721–6.

[64] Chyka PA, Seger D. Position statement: single-dose activated charcoal. J Toxicol Clin Toxicol 1997;35(7):721–41.

[65] Molly DW, Penner SB, Rabson J, et al. Use of sodium bicarbonate to treat tricyclic antidepressant induced arrhythmias in a patient with alkalosis. Can Med Assoc J 1984;130: 1457–9.

[66] Shannon M, Liebelt EL. Toxicology reviews: targeted management strategies for cardiovascular toxicity from tricyclic antidepressant overdose: the pivotal role for alkalinization and sodium loading. Pediatr Emerg Care 1998;14:293–8.

[67] Donovan JW, Akhtar J. Salicylates. In: Ford MD, Delaney KA, Ling LJ, et al, editors. Clinical toxicology. 1st edition. Philadelphia: WB Saunders; 2001. p. 275–80.

[68] Parker D, Martinez C, Stanley C, et al. The analysis of methyl salicylates and salicylic acid from Chinese herbal medicine ingestion. J Anal Toxicol 2004;28(3):214–6.

[69] Bell AJ, Duggan G. Acute methyl salicylate toxicity complicating herbal skin treatment for psoriasis. Emerg Med (Fremantle) 2002;14(2):188–90.

[70] Chan TY, Lee KK, Chan AY, et al. Poisoning due to Chinese proprietary medicines. Hum Exp Toxicol 1995;14(5):434–6.

[71] Levy G. Pharmacokinetics of salicylate elimination in man. J Pharm Sci 1965;54:959–67.

[72] Curry SC. Salicylates. In: Brent J, Wallace KL, Burkhart KK, et al, editors. Critical care toxicology. 1st edition. Philadelphia: Mosby; 2005. p. 621–30.

[73] Seger DL, Murray L. Aspirin and nonsteroidal agents. In: Marx JA, Hockberger RS, Walls RM, Adams J, Barkin RM, Barsan WG, et al, editors. Rosen's Emergency Medicine: Concepts and Clinical Practice. 5th edition. Philadelphia: Mosby; 2002. p. 2076–81.

[74] Dugandzic RM, Tierney MG, Dickinson GE, Dolan MC, McKnight DR. Evaluation of the validity of the Done nomogram in the management of acute salicylate intoxication. Ann Emerg Med 1989;18(11):1186–90.

[75] Fox GN. Hypocalcemia complicating bicarbonate therapy for salicylate poisoning. West J Med 1984;141(1):108–9.

[76] Reid IR. Transient hypercalcemia following overdoses of soluble aspirin tablets. Aust N Z Med 1985;15(3):364.

[77] Proudfoot AT, Krenzelok EP, Vale JA. Position paper on urine alkalinization. J Toxicol Clin Toxicol 2004;42(1):1–26.

[78] Blatman S. Narcotic poisoning of children through accidental ingestion of methadone and in utero. Pediatrics 1974;54(3):329–32.

[79] Kleinschmidt KC, Wainscott M, Ford MD. Opioids. In: Ford MD, Delaney KA, Ling LJ, Erickson T, editors. Clinical Toxicology. 1st edition. Philadelphia: WB Saunders; 2001. p. 627–39.

[80] Erickson TB. Opioids. In: Erickson TB, Aherns WR, Aks SE, Baum CR, Ling LJ, editors. Pediatric Toxicology: Diagnosis and Management of the Poisoned Child. New York: McGraw-Hill; 2005. p. 409–15.

[81] Leblanc A, Benbrick N, Moreau MH. Methadone poisoning in a 1-year-old child treated by continuous infusion of naloxone. Arch Pediatr 2002;9(7):694–6.

[82] Kelly AM, Kerr D, Dietze P, Patrick I, Walker T, Koutsogiannis Z. Randomised trial of intranasal versus intramuscular naloxone in prehospital treatment for suspected opioid overdose. Med J Aust 2005;182(1):24–7.

[83] Mycyk MB, Szyszko AL, Aks SE. Nebulized naloxone gently and effectively reverses methadone intoxication. J Emerg Med 2003;24(2):185–7.

[84] Chumpa A, Kaplan RL, Burns MM, Shannon MW. Nalmefene for elective reversal of procedural sedation in children. Am J Emerg Med 2001;19(7):545–8.

[85] Watson WA, Steele MT, Muelleman RL, Rush MD. Opioid toxicity recurrence after an initial response to naloxone. Clin Toxicol 1998;36(1–2):11–7.

Index

Note: Page numbers of article titles are in **boldface** type.

A

Abdominal trauma, **243–256**
disposition in, 253–254
epidemiology of, 243
hepatic, 250–251, 254–255
history in, 244–245
hospital stay in, 254–255
injuries associated with, 245–246
intestinal, 252–253
laboratory tests in, 246–250
mechanism of injury in, 244
pancreatic, 253
physical examination in, 245–246
renal, 253
splenic, 251–252, 254–255

Abscess, peritonsillar, 223

Absence seizures, 258

Acetohexamide, toxic ingestion of, 294

Acidosis, metabolic
in methanol ingestion, 301
in salicylate ingestion, 307

Activated charcoal, for toxic ingestions
clonidine, 304
opioids, 311
salicylates, 308
sulfonylureas, 295

Acyclovir
for herpetic gingivostomatitis, 204
for neonatal herpes, 173–174

Alanine aminotransferase, in abdominal
trauma, 247–249

Albuterol, for bronchiolitis, 228

Alcohols, ingestion of, 298–303

American Academy of Pediatrics, sedation
guidelines of, 280–281

American Association for the Surgery of
Trauma
liver injury scale of, 251
splenic injury scale of, 251–252

American Society of Anesthesiologists,
physical status classification of, 287

Amitriptyline, toxic ingestion of, 305–307

Amlodipine, toxic ingestion of, 297

Amoxicillin
for bacteremia, 178
for otitis media, 198
for pneumonia, 182
for sinusitis, 203

Amoxicillin-clavulanate
for otitis media, 198
for sinusitis, 203

Ampicillin, for fever without source, 173

Ampicillin-sulbactam, for epiglottitis, 220

Amylase, in abdominal trauma, 250

Analgesia, procedural. *See* Procedural sedation
and analgesia.

Antibiotics
for deep neck space infections, 222
for otitis externa, 196
for otitis media, 198–199

Anticholinergic toxidrome, in antidepressant
ingestion, 305

Antidepressants, toxic ingestion of, 305–307

Antifreeze, ingestion of, 298–303

Anxiolysis, 279

Aspartate aminotransferase, in abdominal
trauma, 247–249

Aspergillus, in otitis externa, 196

Aspirin, toxic ingestion of, 307–309

Atonic seizures, 258

Atypical pneumonia, 228

Auditory canal, inflammation of, 195–197

Avulsion injuries, of tooth, 209–210

0031-3955/06/$ – see front matter © 2006 Elsevier Inc. All rights reserved.
doi:10.1016/S0031-3955(06)00043-5

Croup, 218–219

Crown fractures, 207–208

Culture
blood
in fever without source, 173, 180
in pneumonia, 232
sputum, in pneumonia, 232
throat, in streptococcal pharyngitis,
216–217
urine, in fever without source, 173, 181

D

Deadly ingestions, **293–315**
alcohols, 298–303
calcium channel antagonists, 296–298
clonidine, 303–305
opioids, 309–310
salicylates, 307–309
sulfonylureas, 293–296
tricyclic antidepressants, 305–307

Deep sedation, definition of, 280

Dental trauma, 205–210
anatomic considerations in, 206
avulsion, 209–210
epidemiology of, 205
fractures, 207–208
in abuse, 205
luxation, 208–209
physical examination in, 206–207
radiography in, 207

Dexamethasone
for croup, 218–219
for streptococcal pharyngitis, 217

Diazepam, for seizures, 265, 275

Diet, ketogenic, for seizures, 271

Diltiazem, toxic ingestion of, 297

Diphenhydramine
for herpetic gingivostomatitis, 204
for procedural sedation and analgesia,
283, 285

Dopamine, for clonidine ingestion, 304

Dystonia, versus seizures, 261

E

Ear
foreign bodies in, 199–200
inflammation/infection of
external, 195–197
middle, 197–199

Electroencephalography, in seizures, 264,
271–272

Ellis classification, of tooth fractures, 207–208

Emergency treatment
of abdominal trauma, **243–256**
of airway infections, **215–242**
of deadly ingestions, **293–315**
of ear, nose, and throat conditions,
195–214
of fever without source, **167–194**
of seizures, **257–277**
procedural sedation and analgesia for,
279–292

Empyema, in pneumonia, 226, 233

End-tidal carbon dioxide, monitoring of, in
procedural sedation, 281

Epiglottitis, 219–220

Epilepsy, definition of, 257

Epinephrine
for bronchiolitis, 227
for croup, 218–219
for epistaxis, 201

Epistaxis, 200–201

Epstein-Barr virus infections, splenic rupture
in, 252

Erythromycin
for *Chlamydia trachomatis*
pneumonia, 229
for pertussis, 230

Escherichia coli, in fever without source, 172

Ethanol, ingestion of, 298–303

Ethosuximide, for seizures, 266, 269

Ethylene glycol, ingestion of, 298–303

Etomidate, for procedural sedation and
analgesia, 283, 285

Extrusion injury, of tooth, 209

F

Fasting, for procedural sedation, 288–289

Felbamate, for seizures, 266, 269–270

Felodipine, toxic ingestion of, 297

Fentanyl, for procedural sedation and
analgesia, 282, 284–285

Fever
seizures in, 273–275
without source, in children 0 to 36
months, **167–194**
age-specific considerations in, 171
algorithm for, 184, 186

Somnambulism, 262

Spasms, infantile, 259

Spasmus nutans, versus seizures, 262

Spleen, trauma to, 251–252, 254–255

Sputum culture, in pneumonia, 232

Staphylococcus, in epiglottitis, 219

Staphylococcus aureus, in pneumonia, 226

Status epilepticus
    definition of, 257
    treatment of, 264–267

Steeple sign, in croup, 218

Streptococci
    group A, in pharyngitis, 216–217
    group B, in fever without source, 172
    in epiglottitis, 219

Streptococcus pneumoniae
    in bacteremia, 177–179
    in fever without source, 181–182
      epidemiology of, 168–170
      in neonates, 172–173
      in older infants and toddlers, 177–179
      in young infants, 175
    in otitis media, 198
    in pneumonia, 181–182, 225–227
    vaccine for, 168–170, 182–183

Stridor, in croup, 218

Subluxation, of tooth, 208

Sulfonylureas, toxic ingestion of, 293–296

Supraglottitis, 219–220

Swimmer's ear, 195–197

T

Tachycardia, due to calcium channel antagonists, 297

Teeth, injury of. *See* Dental trauma.

Thermal cautery, for epistaxis, 201

Thiamine, for ethylene glycol ingestion, 302

Throat, infections of, 204–205, 216–217

Throat culture, in streptococcal pharyngitis, 216–217

Tiagabine, for seizures, 266, 270

Tics, versus seizures, 261

Tolazamide, toxic ingestion of, 294

Tonic-clonic seizures, 258

Tonsillitis, 216–217, 223

Topiramate, for seizures, 266, 270, 273

Toxic ingestions. *See* Deadly ingestions.

Transfusion, for abdominal trauma, 254

Trauma
    abdominal. *See* Abdominal trauma.
    dental. *See* Dental trauma.

Tricyclic antidepressants, toxic ingestion of, 305–307

Trimethoprim-sulfamethoxazole, for pertussis, 230

"Tripod position," in epiglottitis, 219–220

U

Ultrasonography, in deep neck space infections, 222

Urinalysis
    in abdominal trauma, 247–249
    in fever without source, 173, 181

Urinary tract infections, fever in
    in older infants and toddlers, 180–181, 186
    in young infants, 176

Urine culture, in fever without source, 173, 181

V

Vaccines, *Streptococcus pneumoniae,* 168–170, 182–183

Valproic acid, for seizures, 266, 269

Vancomycin, for streptococcal pneumonia, 226

Verapamil, toxic ingestion of, 297

Vigabatrin, for seizures, 266, 270

Viral infections
    in neonates, 173–174
    oropharyngeal, 204–205
    pharyngotonsillar, 216
    pneumonia, 225

Visual loss, in methanol ingestion, 301

W

West's syndrome, 259

Z

Zonisamide, for seizures, 266, 271, 273

the bleeding is controlled) and to keep the head elevated but not hyperextended to avoid aspiration of the blood [2] . Usually only 5 to 10 minutes is required to stop the bleeding. A piece of gauze soaked with a nasal decongestant spray, epinephrine at a ratio of 1:10,000, or phenylephrine and placed in the affected nostril may also be helpful to induce localized vasoconstriction. If bleeding cannot be controlled with these simple measures, then transfer to an emergency department is required.

The emergency department initial evaluation of the patient with epistaxis involves the assessment of the airway, breathing, and circulation (ABC). A posterior bleed is more likely than an anterior bleed to cause airway compromise or blood aspiration and may rarely require intubation to protect the airway. Hemodynamic instability must be evaluated and quickly addressed. Once cardiopulmonary stability has been established, the physical examination should include a nasal examination with a good light source and a handheld nasal speculum. The nasal cavity should first be cleared of clots with suction and forceps to allow visualization of the nasal mucosa and evaluation of obvious sources of bleeding [15].

If an anterior source of bleeding is identified and the bleeding is active, cautery may be helpful after localized anesthesia and topical vasoconstriction, using either silver nitrate sticks or thermal cautery. Cautery causes injury to the nasal mucosa, resulting in coagulation or blood vessel constriction to effect cessation of the bleeding [15]. Care must be taken when cauterizing a bleed to prevent damage to surrounding structures and perforation of the nasal septum. Anterior bleeding that is unresponsive to cautery may require anterior nasal packing with petroleum jelly (Vasoline) gauze strips or a commercial packing that expands when it becomes wet to tamponade the bleeding vessel. Packing should be preceded by the application of local anesthesia and nasal decongestants [15]. The removal of packing and a reevaluation can take place after 15 to 30 minutes.

The failure to identify an anterior source of bleeding is a possible indication of posterior bleeding. Posterior bleeding may be indicated by hemoptysis, hematemesis, or blood in the posterior pharynx [17]. Posterior epistaxis is less amenable to cautery secondary to the quantity of bleeding and often requires posterior nasal packing or epistaxis balloons [15]. These patients should be managed in conjunction with a specialist and usually require admission to the hospital because of the risk of hypoxia or respiratory compromise. In addition, children with a posterior nasal packing or epistaxis balloon should be treated with a course of antibiotics that provides staphylococcal and streptococcal coverage to decrease the incidence of sinusitis or toxic shock syndrome.

Sinusitis

Sinusitis is a relatively common form of upper respiratory tract infection in the pediatric population. The challenge for the emergency pediatric physician is to distinguish among an uncomplicated viral or allergic rhinosinusitis and acute, subacute, and chronic bacterial sinusitis. The classic presenting symptoms of sinusitis in adults and teenage patients with mature sinuses are rarely present in the preadolescent patient.

Sinus development starts in utero and continues through the teenage years. The maxillary and ethmoid sinuses form during the third to fourth months of gestation and are the only sinuses present at birth. The frontal sinus begins to develop by 1 to 2 years of age from an anterior ethmoid cell and migrates to a supraorbital position. The frontal sinus is not seen radiologically until approximately age 5 or 6. By the early teenage years, the sinuses have enlarged to their adult capacity.

The maxillary, frontal, and anterior ethmoid sinuses drain through ostia into the middle meatus, beneath the middle turbinate in the nose. The outflow tract of the maxillary sinus is located on the upper medial wall of the sinus, which makes drainage by gravity difficult and predisposes patients to infection. The ethmoid sinuses are composed of multiple individual air cells that each drain through their own narrow ostia. These narrow tracts may be obstructed by thick secretions or mucosal inflammation, resulting in infection of the ethmoid sinuses. The frontal and sphenoid sinuses are, less commonly, primary sites of infection; however, they may be affected in pansinusitis, and infection may spread from them to the orbit or central nervous system.

Acute bacterial sinusitis

The classic presenting symptoms for acute bacterial sinusitis in the adult population (including fever, headache, facial pain, tenderness, and facial edema) are less common in children. Fever, if present, is often low grade. Nasal discharge is a common symptom, but the quality of nasal discharge varies from thin and clear to thick and purulent. Patients often have cough, although it is not always described as productive. Cough may be present in the daytime, although it is often worse at night or when lying supinely during naps.

In the pediatric patient, two qualities can help distinguish between a viral rhinosinusitis and an acute bacterial sinusitis:

- Persistence of symptoms: Upper respiratory tract infections with symptoms that last more than 10 days, without any improvement, are more likely to represent bacterial sinusitis [18]. Most uncomplicated viral infections last approximately 5 to 7 days, and if not resolved by the tenth day, they have at least shown significant improvement.
- Increased severity of symptoms: Severe symptoms are defined as the combination of high fever ($\geq 39°C$ [$\geq 102°F$]) and purulent nasal discharge or classic symptoms of acute sinusitis such as facial swelling and pain [18,19]. The presence of high fever and purulent nasal discharge lasting for at least 3 to 4 days indicate a likely bacterial sinusitis. Patients with viral nasosinusitis may have fever, but it is usually associated with constitutional

symptoms in the early or prodromal phase of illness. Purulent nasal discharge may also develop in patients with viral infections, but it usually occurs later in the course of illness and clears to a watery or mucoid consistency before resolution.

Subacute and chronic bacterial sinusitis

The duration of symptoms of more than 30 days separates acute from subacute or chronic bacterial sinusitis. Nasal congestion (as opposed to discharge) and cough are the most common respiratory symptoms. Sore throat may be present from constant mouth breathing. Headache is a less common symptom, and fever is extremely rare [18].

Diagnostic imaging

Plain radiographs, including the Waters (occipitofrontal), Caldwell (angled posteroanterior), and lateral views, have traditionally been used to aid in diagnosing sinusitis. Radiographic findings that suggest a diagnosis of sinusitis (in the presence of appropriate clinical symptoms) include diffuse opacification, mucosal thickening (≥ 4 mm), or air-fluid levels [20]. CT scanning of the sinuses has been the gold standard for diagnosis. Because of the speed and increased accessibility of CT scanners in the emergency department, sinus CT scanning is becoming the first-line choice for radiographic diagnosis of sinusitis.

Treatment

Sinusitis does have a high spontaneous cure rate, but antibiotics remain a mainstay of treatment in any pediatric practice [21]. The first-line therapy for uncomplicated acute bacterial sinusitis is high-dose amoxicillin, although with emerging resistance patterns in certain areas, there are a number of other therapeutic options. Recommendations on the choice of antibiotic therapy are similar to those for otitis media infection.

Initial treatment with an antibiotic with broader coverage, such as amoxicillin-clavulanate or cefuroxime, is warranted in patients who show no improvement on amoxicillin or who have been treated with amoxicillin within the previous month, in locations with a high prevalence of β-lactamase-producing *H influenzae*, in the presence of frontal or sphenoid sinusitis or complicated ethmoidal sinusitis, or with a diagnosis of subacute or chronic sinusitis. In areas with a high frequency of infection with penicillin- and cephalosporin-resistant pneumococci, other antibiotics are available, including azithromycin, trimethoprim-sulfamethoxazole, and clindamycin. Antibiotic choices should be guided by culture and sensitivities when available. The duration of treatment is usually 10 to 14 days. Most patients show improvement within 3 to 4 days, and the guidelines recommendation continuing treatment for 7 days after the patient is asymptomatic [18].

Oral cavity lesions

Herpes simplex virus

The most common presentation of primary herpes simplex virus (HSV) infection in young children is herpetic gingivostomatitis. It is seen most often in children ages 6 months to 5 years. Because of its significant discomfort and disturbing appearance, it regularly triggers physician and emergency department visits. HSV is transmitted through infectious saliva and has an incubation period of 2 to 12 days, with a mean of 4 days. Viral shedding, however, can occur from 7 days to as long as 3 weeks or more after clinical infection [22]. The primary infection may present with associated flu-like symptoms, including an abrupt onset of high fever, irritability, and malaise. Oral findings include erythematous, edematous, and friable gingivae as well as oral and perioral clusters of vesicles, which coalesce to form large, painful ulcers. Symptoms usually last less than 1 week but may continue for up to 21 days [23].

HSV is usually diagnosed clinically, although confirmation is possible by viral culture of the vesicular fluid or by the identification of multinucleated giant cells on a Tzanck smear from the base of the lesions. The treatment of herpetic gingivostomatitis is primarily supportive. Analgesics and antipyretics (such as acetaminophen and ibuprofen) can be used. In more severe cases, oral opiates may be necessary. Topical anesthetics such as diphenhydramine syrup mixed in a 1:1 solution with magnesia hydroxide (Maalox) may be applied to the affected mucosa every 2 hours [24]. A small amount of the solution may be painted on the lesions of younger children. Older children may be instructed to spit out the solution after rinsing but should not swallow it. Although viscous lidocaine is commonly included in this topical solution, it should be avoided because of its potential for toxicity. Other nonprescription medications that can be used topically as a barrier to irritants include zilactin, docosanol (Abreva), and ORA-5, although their use is off-label in children [24].

Because of the significant pain associated with HSV lesions, children are at risk of dehydration from decreased oral intake. Oral fluid administration should be highly encouraged. Parents should be advised to give children oral fluids in the form of popsicles or ice, which soothe the oral lesions and are therefore more readily consumed.

Antiviral therapy may be helpful for the treatment of oral HSV disease if it is started within 72 hours of the onset of lesions [25]. Patients treated early with acyclovir have a shorter duration of lesions, earlier resolution of fever and extraoral lesions, a shorter duration of poor oral intake, and decreased viral shedding [26]. Topical acyclovir has no role in the treatment of primary oral HSV